Research on
Infectious Diseases

at
The University of Maryland
School of Medicine & Hospital
A Global Experience
1807 to 2000

EDITED BY THEODORE E. WOODWARD, M.D.

With contributions by Clyde, Edelman, Gallo, Greisman,
Hornick, Levine, McCrumb, Parker, Schimpff,
Strickland, Togo, Warren, Wisseman and Woodward

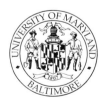

In Collaboration with the University of Maryland
School of Medicine and the Medical Alumni Association, Baltimore

The University of Maryland School of Medicine and the
Medical Alumni Association of the University of Maryland, Inc.
522 West Lombard Street
Baltimore, Maryland 21201

Printed in the United States of America

*This history is dedicated with pride and esteem
to those many alumni, house officers,
faculty members (past and present), professional and
military colleagues, and civilian volunteers.
It is a culmination of their devotion, enthusiasm, courage,
and comprehensive studies on detection, treatment, and
prevention of conventional and tropical infectious diseases
throughout the world.*

CONTENTS

CONTRIBUTORS

David Clyde, M.D., Ph.D.   Professor of Medicine, Head,
                                International Health Program,
                                Director, Program on Malaria,
                                Senior Malariologist, WHO

Robert Edelman, M.D.   Professor of Medicine, Geographic
                                Medicine, Associate Director,
                                Center, Vaccine Development

Robert C. Gallo, M.D.   Professor of Medicine, Director,
                                Institute of Human Virology

Sheldon E. Greisman, M.D.   Professor of Medicine, Physiology

Richard B. Hornick, M.D.   Professor of Medicine, Head,
                                Division of Infectious Diseases

Myron M. Levine, M.D.,   Professor of Medicine, Geographic
  DTPH   Medicine, Pediatrics, Director,
                                Center, Vaccine Development
                                (C.V.D.)

Robert T. Parker, M.D.	Associate Professor of Medicine, Head, Division of Infectious Diseases
Stephen C. Schimpff, M.D.	Professor of Medicine, Head, Division of Infectious Diseases, CEO University of Maryland Health System
Jennifer Schorr	Public Affairs Coordinator, Institute of Human Virology
G. Thomas Strickland, M.D., Ph.D.	Director, International Health Program
Yasushi Togo, M.D.	Assistant Professor of Medicine, Head, Diagnostic Virology, Section Head, Research and Development, Merck & Co. Tokyo, Japan
John W. Warren, M.D.	Professor of Medicine, Head, Division of Infectious Diseases
Theodore E. Woodward, M.D.	Professor of Medicine, Emeritus, 1st Director, Division of Infectious Diseases

PREFACE

For almost two centuries, University of Maryland Medical School faculty members, alumni, hospital attending physicians, and medical students were very active in studying and contributing new knowledge to the field of infectious diseases. This history attempts to describe these timely contributions with focus on the various clinical manifestations, epidemiologic characteristics, practical means of confirmation of diagnoses through application of available and new laboratory techniques, the relevant mechanisms of pathologic physiology, and effective specific new forms of treatment. Baltimore, as a major port of the eastern United States, provided opportunities to cope with serious human infections imported from South America, Europe, Asia, Africa, and Far Eastern ports. Due to the close proximity of several tropical islands to the United States, tropical medicine in the early days and even today has proven to be a significant component of the practicing physician's daily problems.

Much of the world was literally the working laboratory for those professionals who conceived and performed the various investigative studies. These were not "fly by night" brief visits to foreign sites, but involved sufficient time periods to meet and associate with foreign colleagues, and collect epidemiologic, clinical, and laboratory information in the locally established medical centers. Before such collaborative work could be consummated, arrangements were made with the health ministries of the various foreign countries to be visited. Moreover, during the mid and late 20th century, much of the work had the full collaboration, sponsorship, and resource assistance from the U.S. Department of Defense and the National Institutes of Health of the Public Health Service.

The foreign sites which collaborated with the University of Maryland School of Medicine and Hospital were Jamaica, Puerto Rico, Peru, Chile, Panama, Italy, Greece, Morocco, Algeria, Egypt, Iran, India, East and West Pakistan, Japan, Korea, Philippines, Thailand, Vietnam, Malaysia, New Guinea, Singapore, and Indonesia.

The infectious diseases categories comprising this longstanding work were broad and included the following: Rickettsial diseases (epidemic, murine, and scrub typhus; Rocky Mountain spotted fever; Q fever), enteric diseases (typhoid fever, cholera, *Escherichia coli* infections, dysentery, amoebic and bacillary), insect-borne infections, yellow fever, dengue, viral encephalitis, bacterial infections (meningitis, septicemia, plague, tularemia, endocarditis), common viral diseases (influenza, mumps, measles, varicella, variola, sandfly fever, Coxsackie disease, chlamydia, primary atypical pneumonia).

Naturally we are proud of Fred McCrumb, Robert Parker, Yash Togo, Richard Hornick, Steven Schimpff, Myron Levine, Robert Edelman, Robert Gallo, Thomas Strickland, and their colleagues, not only for their important contributions to this voluminous work, but for having taken time from their busy schedules to prepare their respective chapters.

Gratitude and sincere thanks are expressed in memory of Mrs. Sarah Whitehurst, a prominent Marylander and national public servant. Mrs. Whitehurst, a graduate of the University of Maryland Nursing School, became an important contributing member of the University of Maryland Board of Regents serving under several presidents. While traveling in the western United States, she developed an acute febrile illness with a rash, thought initially by her physician to be Rocky Mountain spotted fever. She was very seriously ill and received devoted expert care by the professional medical and nursing staff of the hospital. She recovered fully after experiencing an extremely severe type of neoplasm. Her productive life continued for a number of years. She and her husband, Mr. John Whitehurst, were very generous in bequeathing funds to the nursing school and hospital for educational and research objectives. These funds have helped defray the necessary costs for publication of this book.

ACKNOWLEDGMENT

Grateful appreciation is expressed to numerous persons to whom I am sincerely indebted. They are: Mrs. Celeste Marousek, Mrs. Joyce Krebner, Mrs. Wanda Johnson, Mrs. Peggy Riley, Mrs. Harriet Kerr, and Ms. Molly Lutz, who prepared various sections of the manuscript. Mrs. Marousek and Mrs. Krebner carefully retyped the final draft. Some of the initial sections were typed by my long-time secretary, Mrs. Carol Young. I am indebted and grateful for their expert help.

Photographs were carefully prepared for publication by the Medical Media Department of the VA Medical Center. Mr. Stephen A. Johnston and his staff at Brushwood Graphics, Inc., in collaboration with Ms. Betsy Winship of Stoney Run Publishing Services, carefully edited the manuscript and arranged the descriptive material and photographs.

Mr. Larry R. Pitrof, Executive Director of the Maryland Medical Alumni Association and Drs. Frank M. Calia and Philip A. Mackowiak of the Department of Medicine gave assistance in recalling old events as well as editorial assistance. Naturally, we are beholden to each of the co-authors, who, in spite of their many responsibilities, prepared their individual, informative sections. My wife, Celeste, provided stimulus, encouragement and support as well as a careful check of my spelling and recall of dates of old events.

T.E.W.

1

INTRODUCTION
Infectious Diseases in Colonial America

Theodore E. Woodward, M.D.

Infectious diseases ravaged the early colonies and caused untold numbers of deaths and serious illnesses. In a way, it can be said that the Europeans practiced unpremeditated biological warfare against the early Americans since they brought most of the diseases with them. There is no question that the white man's diseases of Europe contributed to the elimination of the Native American population in early America.

Smallpox, yellow fever, and diphtheria often struck suddenly in epidemic proportions and caused panic and death. The respiratory infections, particularly the common cold, influenza, pleurisy, and pneumonia, ranked about third in the cause of suffering and death. Dysentery and malaria were less alarming in their impact; however, they became chronic and probably were responsible for both social and economic losses.

The common childhood diseases (measles, pertussis, and mumps) probably, overall, caused the largest number of deaths. Also the enteric infections, particularly dysentery and typhoid fever, had high marks for disability. Cholera came a little later and often struck with lightning speed, particularly in the Eastern cities, before it spread to the Midwest and down the Mississippi. By the mid 1700s, 43% of the new missionaries had either died or resigned and returned to Europe because of the impact and threat of infections.

Smallpox, one of the major problems, was ultimately controlled with the procedure of variolation which was practiced in America until Jennerian vaccination became available. Diphtheria (or "putrid" sore throat of children) and scarlet fever were actually more important than the other childhood diseases. Yellow fever was the most malignant of all the scourges and caused general havoc.

As mentioned previously, more Native Americans died of white man's diseases than from weaponry. Smallpox was the worst offender for them, and epidemic louse-borne typhus fever was not far behind.

Better living conditions and the practice of variolation in the late 18th century helped reduce the incidence and spread of infections. By the early and mid-19th century, things were much better.[1]

BRIEF HISTORICAL SYNOPSIS
OF SPECIFIC CHEMOTHERAPY

The painfully acquired knowledge of specific remedies for infectious diseases began with quinine, mercury, antimony, emetine, and the salicylates, which were somewhat effective chiefly against the larger infectious agents, the protozoa, especially the plasmodia of malaria and the spirochetes, particularly treponema pallidum. Development of the sulfonamides made bacteria vulnerable, in particular, the Gram-positive organisms, especially the coccal groups. Introduction of the antibiotics, with penicillin in the forefront, further extended the field of specific medication, without however, showing much effect upon those diseases caused by the Gram-negative group of bacilli. Certain of the Gram-negative organisms began to yield with streptomycin, including mycobacterium tuberculosis. The range of this drug extended to the agents of plague, tularemia, and brucellosis. Streptomycin's effect on the still smaller group of infectious agents, the rickettsia and viruses, was slight and of no clinical significance. The two new broad-spectrum antibiotics introduced in 1948,

Chloromycetin and Aureomycin, not only successfully combated certain important human infections caused by Gram-negative bacilli as well as Gram-positive bacteria, but showed themselves to be highly specific for all members of the rickettsial group. Furthermore, they were effective for a few of the viral-like agents of disease (e.g., lymphopathia venereum and psittacosis). The defenses of the true viruses were now broached.

ESTABLISHMENT OF FIRST CLINICAL DIAGNOSTIC LABORATORY

Charles E. Simon was born in Baltimore on September 23, 1866, but obtained his primary education in Germany. When his family returned to America, he studied chemistry at the Johns Hopkins University and received his B.A. degree from the University of Pennsylvania in 1888. His degree in medicine was awarded by the University of Maryland in 1890. After his graduation, he came under the tutelage of William Osler and, later, William Welch, who encouraged his further training in physiologic chemistry in France and Germany. He then practiced medicine in Baltimore, specializing primarily in gastrointestinal diseases.

Dr. Simon established the first available diagnostic laboratory in an abandoned shed. His aim was to assist physicians in establishing a specific diagnosis of illness. Dr. Welch helped him acquire fellowship and research funds with Abraham Flexner's support from the Rockefeller Institute. The first grant was awarded to him in 1907.

Using experimental animal models and microscopic staining procedures, he first worked on detecting antibodies in various types of cancer. Later he identified various inclusions from tissues of infectious diseases, such as measles, varicella, variola, and filterable viruses, such as herpes,

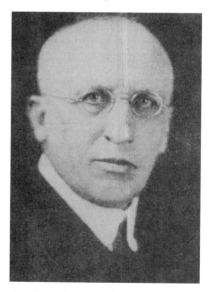

Charles E. Simon, M.D.

trachoma, and influenza. Simon developed a national reputation as an authority on clinical diagnosis and as a founder of the discipline of virology. These capabilities culminated in his appointment at the College of Physicians and Surgeons of Baltimore (Mercy Hospital). He held appointments as Professor of Clinical Pathology and Experimental Medicine simultaneously at the College of Physicians and Surgeons and the University of Maryland School of Medicine. These two schools merged in 1915. He was a thorough and dedicated teacher who linked laboratory instruction with bedside examinations in hospitals. Students and physicians who studied under him became thoroughly grounded in clinical diagnosis.

Dr. Simon remained at the University of Maryland until 1919 when he left because of rather prevalent anti-German sentiments. From 1919 to 1920, he became a volunteer assistant at the Johns Hopkins School of Public Health and Hygiene. Here he developed the first course in filterable viruses, beginning in 1922. Simon and his assistants, along with special students, published papers on the diagnosis of smallpox and experimental studies of measles, cell inclusions in varicella, the formation of Guarnieri bodies, and the origin of malignant growth. The unit which he organized was probably the first formal course in laboratory filterable viruses. It became a source of professionals trained in this special new field. Many of Simon's students went to other institutions where they established the *American Journal of Hygiene* for publication of technical research in public health and preventive medicine. William H. Welch was editor, and Simon was the managing editor. Simon died on November 8, 1927. His legacy described by William H. Howell, Dean of the School of Hygiene, was "the development of the subject of filterable viruses throughout the country, and [he has] added greatly to the reputation and influence of this school as a center of research in preventive medicine."[2]

In the following pages, other contributions to detection, prevention, treatment, and pathophysiologic understanding of major infectious diseases made by University of Maryland faculty members and its associated practitioners are described. Through their dedicated work and remarkable achievements, great progress in public health was made which extended over two centuries.

REFERENCES

1. Duffy J. Epidemics in Colonial America. Louisiana State University Press: Baton Rouge, 1953.

2. Harvey AM. Pioneer American virologist—Charles E. Simon. Johns Hopkins Med Bull 1978;142:161–186.

2

Yellow Fever

Theodore E. Woodward, M.D.

Benjamin Rush long held the view that yellow fever became contagious under unfavorable conditions, and the writings on this disease contain constant references to the effect of heat, moisture, and organic decomposition on the spread of the disease. After investigating the Philadelphia outbreak of 1793, Rush declared in the following year that it originated from some putrid coffee that had been discharged from a vessel.

Nathaniel Potter, a former private pupil of Rush during the epidemic in Philadelphia in 1793, returned to Baltimore later that year and attended patients there and in Caroline County of the Eastern Shore of Maryland. His keen clinical and epidemiologic observations convinced him that yellow fever was not contagious between persons. He communicated by letter with his old teacher on August 20, 1793 and again on October 28, 1793. Potter detailed the circumstances of the epidemic in Caroline County and stated:

> Those various forms of bilious fever, unquestionably owe their existence to the putrefaction of matters on the surface of the earth, after an uncommonly wet spring, followed by the driest and hottest

summer that can be remembered by the oldest inhabitants of the county. Whatsoever may be the result of controversy so warmly agitated in your city, respecting the contagion of yellow fever; the epidemic has no pretensions to that character, in any of its forms. The dysenteric form is considered contagious by popular consent, but (mejudice) is no more entitled to the epithet contagious, than the remittent or intermittent fevers. With all possible deference to your superior judgment, I cannot prevail upon myself to believe that any fever, arising from vegetable decomposition, is contagious. The origin you have assigned to the epidemick fever of your city is the only one that is physically possible, and therefore, you place your adversaries on equal ground with you, by acknowledging the fever contagious. Deny the existence of contagion as unphilosophical, and you've cut them off from every resource. If we admit one of the fevers from marsh effluvia to be contagious, we are bound (a priore), to admit them all to be so; intermittent, remittent, and dysenteric.[1]

Potter, who considered himself the only person in America to deny the contagion of yellow fever, requested Rush to publish these views in his paper describing the Philadelphia epidemic of 1793. Rush declined the proposal and stated his firm belief, "that all diseases arising from marsh miasmata were contagious in a degree proportional to their malignity, and that the opposite doctrine was utterly untenable" (p. III).[1] Potter, in quoting his views regarding the quarantine laws of Philadelphia against Baltimore, felt "there could not be a more flagrant or more lamentable proof that the framers of these laws were destitute of every ray of knowledge of the true qualities of contagion, than the exemption of smallpox from the provision of their quarantine laws. That disease which assails our bodies through every sense but one, whose concentrated poison can be preserved for years, which ocular demonstration has proved to have been transported to every part of the commercial world, is permitted to scourge mankind, while we are legislating against a phantom, against a superstition, against a *campaign* of fear and imagination, heightened by a mixture of the marvelous, as fabulous as any of the tales comprehended within the complicated machinery of the heathen mythology. The visions of contagion stand on a parallel with the calculations of judicial astrology, solemn exorcisms, enchanted castles, and the spells of wizards and witches. The age of chivalry is not gone" (p. 113).[1]

Thus, Potter protested the views of his former tutor, Benjamin Rush. Potter, to prove his conviction went to the extremes of soaking towels in the "perspirable" matter of a patient with yellow fever whom he attended on September 20, 1797. He bound it about his head, retired, and reported that in spite of "extreme nauseous fetor," he experienced transient sickness but slept until 7 o'clock a.m. There was no later incapacitation. In 1798, Potter inoculated himself with "perspirable matter" from a patient with yellow fever during the last stages. From other malignant cases, he took suppurative matter from inguinal buboes and inoculated himself on October 11, 1798. He experienced only local redness at the inoculating site. Potter's courageous but ill-conceived self-studies really proved nothing since he was either resistant (immune) because of a prior attack of yellow fever or his test patients did not suffer from the disease or had eliminated the virus from their tissue.

Potter became the first Professor of Medicine at the University of Maryland, taking the Chair in 1807. His classic monograph on yellow fever in 1818 describes his life experiences and those perceptive observations recorded during outbreaks of yellow fever in Maryland.

The first printed denunciation of the contagion of yellow fever was by Potter's colleague, John Beale Davidge, the founder of the University of Maryland School of Medicine, and its Professor of Anatomy and Dean.[2]

Davidge was a general practitioner and a practical epidemiologist. Experiences at Baltimore's Fells and Locust Points in the harbor area convinced him of the noncontagiousness of yellow fever which he published in the *Federal Gazette of Baltimore* on November 30, 1797. This communication was reaffirmed, enlarged, and embodied in a small monograph, published first in 1798 and reprinted in 1813. Potter's and Davidge's clinical descriptions of yellow fever, like other keenly observant clinicians of the colonial era, were remarkably good.

Another Baltimore physician was prophetic in his introductory academic address in 1811 when he predicted a relationship between insects and human illness. John Crawford said: "It is not alone in our fields or our gardens that they commit their ravages, they attack us in our houses, our goods, our furniture, our clothes, our poultry; they devour the grain in our storehouse, they pierce all our woodwork, they do not spare us, even ourselves."

Crawford proposed:

> I shall then proceed to consider the cause of suffering in the animals that are in the nearest connection with us, continue my inquiries through all of the animal tribes down to the smallest insect, as far as the means for information have been within my reach. . . . so with men, the plague, yellow and every other fever and every other disease we experience, must be occasioned by eggs inserted without our knowledge into our bodies.[3,4]

Throughout the 19th century, outbreaks of yellow fever persisted in developing America, obeyed the summer cycle, ceased with the onset of frost, favored southeastern, southern, and gulf coastal cities, and eluded explanation. Cities hardest hit were New York, Philadelphia, Baltimore, Norfolk, Charleston, Memphis, Galveston, and New Orleans. The last yellow fever epidemic in the continental United States was in New Orleans in 1905; there were 3,384 cases and 443 deaths, nearly all in the "old town." The sporadic outbreaks which occurred in Baltimore in 1800, 1808, 1819, 1853, 1854, and 1876 began usually at Locust and Fells Points after ships docked from the Indies. Areas of Baltimore west of Jones Falls and on high ground seemed to possess strange powers of safety.

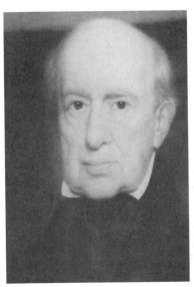

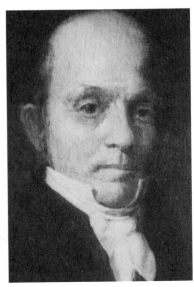

Nathaniel Potter, M.D.   *John B. Davidge, M.D.*

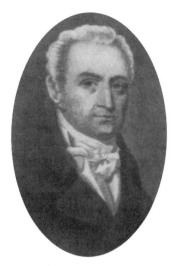

John Crawford, M.D.

The Golden Microbiological Era initiated by Pasteur and Koch in the 1880s, with men like William H. Welch and Theobald Smith in America, helped set the stage for solution of the yellow fever puzzle. Fortified with the observed clinical and epidemiologic facts, scholarly physicians with roots in Philadelphia and Baltimore played major roles.

There are several less acknowledged persons, one an unheralded scholarly epidemiologist and the other a courageous clinical bacteriologist, who merit recognition. Each is an alumnus of the University of Maryland School of Medicine.

Henry Rose Carter is relatively unknown as a participant in the dramatic yellow fever story, yet Walter Reed acknowledged his clue which guided the Reed Commission to success where Carlos Finlay (originator of the mosquito vector concept) had failed. Carter, born in Caroline County, Virginia, fractured his leg after graduation from the University of Virginia, shifted from an engineering career to medicine, enrolled in 1873 at the University

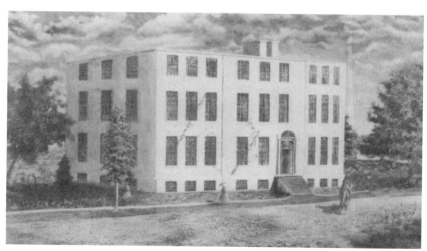

University of Maryland Hospital, 1823 (Baltimore Infirmary)

of Maryland Medical School, and graduated in 1878, at age 26. He interned at its University Hospital and joined the United States Public Health Service with ultimate assignment to the Marine Quarantine Service; his district embraced several islands and ports in the Gulf of Mexico. Skeptically, Carter questioned the 100-year-old explanation that the agent of yellow fever was conveyed by fomites (Miasma), contaminated by direct contact with the primary case. For 20 years, he recorded his observations of outbreaks of yellow fever aboard ships arriving at ports in the Gulf Islands and noted a pattern aboard ships which left South America ports, such as Rio; one or two primary cases occurred within a day or two of embarkation, followed by an interval of two or three weeks and a cluster of new cases. Clustering was not reported by crews whose voyages lasted less than two weeks. No yellow fever occurred among baggage inspectors working in the Gulf district who unpacked and inspected baggage from notorious ports, such as Vera Cruz, Havana, and Santiago. Quarantine records back through 120 years were checked. In 1897, Carter contracted yellow fever and recovered.

In 1898, two years before the dramatic report of the Reed Commission, Carter investigated household outbreaks of yellow fever in Orwood and Taylor, two small towns in northern Mississippi, and concluded that an "extrinsic incubation period" was required for the human transmission of the agent.

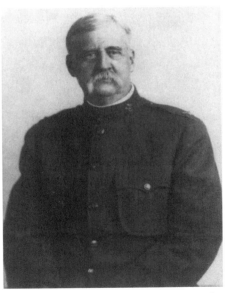

The following observed event from the text of his original paper is a typical example of how Carter validated the case for an extrinsic incubation period. "Mr. S.W.G. of Orwood, was stricken on August 1, remaining in his household for the duration of his illness. Among eight people visiting him between August 6 and

Henry Rose Carter (Courtesy of the National Library of Medicine)

August 17, there were no cases of yellow fever; among 34 people visiting him thereafter, there were 33 cases." Carter concluded: "The material leaving the patient must undergo some changes in the environment before it is capable of infecting another man. The time required for this change is the time of extrinsic incubation."[5]

Transferred to Havana in 1899, to reorganize its quarantine service, Carter met Reed and his team which began its work in June 1900. He kept in close touch with Reed and Jesse Lazear, who were already familiar with his Mississippi studies through reports which he had sent them. Reed, himself, expressed the significance of Carter's work upon the Cuban studies: "You [Carter] must not forget that your work in Mississippi did more to impress me with the importance of an intermediate host than anything else put together." Carter had fixed the extrinsic incubation period at 10 to 17 days; the Reed group set it at 9 to 16 days.

Sir Ronald Ross, who incriminated the anopheline mosquito as the vector of malaria, appreciated the significance of Carter's work and recommended him, along with Finlay, for the 1904 Nobel Prize in Medicine. Recognition and honor were bestowed on Reed, Finlay, and Lazear, but not on Carter or in full measure to the next contributor.

James Carroll, born in Woolwich, England, on June 5, 1855, emigrated to Canada at the age of 15, entered the United States Army, and while a soldier in 1886–1887, began the study of Medicine in New York. He transferred to the University of Maryland School of Medicine and received his degree there in 1891. For two years, he undertook postgraduate work in pathology and bacteriology which included training at the Johns Hopkins Medical School. He met Walter Reed in 1893 during assignment to the Army Medical School in Washington. They were associated for six years before Surgeon-General George Sternberg formed the second Yellow Fever Commission in 1899, with Walter Reed, Director; James Carroll, second in command; and Jesse Lazear and Aristedes Agramonte, who were already in Cuba, as members. Reed and Carroll sailed from New York on June 21, 1900, and reached Havana on June 25. Reed returned to the United States on August 4 with Carroll placed in charge of the field work of this historical drama which incriminated the mosquito. Carroll shouldered the lion's share of work, without which the mission objective may have failed. Based on his strong bacteriologic capability, his initial work with Agramonte disproved Giuseppe Sanarelli's view that *Bacillus icteroides* caused yellow fever. The small group pursued the mosquito concept which Finlay had failed to confirm. They worked amicably with Finlay throughout their trials. Lazear, the team's entomologist, allowed a suitable incubation in mosquitoes after they had been fed on yellow fever patients. On August 27, Lazear placed a mosquito upon Carroll which had been incubated for 12 days. In four days, Carroll suffered a severe, nonfatal attack. This was the first experimentally infected case in history. The views of all noncontagionists, such as Potter and Davidge, were now confirmed.

Later Surgeon-General Sternberg commented that "the incubation in the body of the mosquito was probably Reed's idea; and work along that line caused the first successful case—Carroll's case." Tragically, about two weeks after Carroll's recovery, Lazear died of yellow fever on September 25, 1900.

Carroll continued in charge of the field studies until Reed returned to Cuba, again for a short period from October 3 to October 13, and later directed the studies in which Pvt. Kissinger developed induced yellow fever after being bitten by several mosquitoes which had been contaminated by feeding on patients 15, 19, and 22 days previously. Also, during this period, the classic work in volunteers was performed which showed that clothing, bedding, and discharges of yellow fever patients were not infectious.

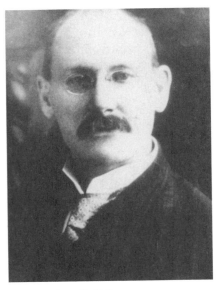

James C. Carroll, M.D.

In the summer of 1901, William H. Welch of the Johns Hopkins University, had suggested the possibility of filterability of the infectious agent to Walter Reed, based on studies of Loeffler and Frosch on foot and mouth disease of cattle.[6]

The use of volunteers for work in Cuba became a sensitive issue, because in 1901, Finlay and his associate, John Guiteras, while conducting vaccine studies in volunteers, independent of the Reed team, encountered two deaths. This alarmed them and the public. Reed, then in Blue Ridge Summit, Pennsylvania, became disturbed by the exaggerated reports which reached him through the press and wrote Carroll on August 23, 1901, who was busy recruiting volunteers and conducting the clinical screening and performing the microbiologic and entomologic studies: "You say 'prospects favorable.' And this leads me to strongly advise against further experiments on humans. Our work has been too good to be marred now by a death. As much as I would like to know whether the filtrate will convey the disease, I shall advise against it."

Carroll now was forced to stand alone. It is clear from the available correspondence between Carroll and Reed at this juncture that the Yellow Fever Commission owes the completion of the final stage of its work to Carroll's wisdom and self-reliance.

In all of the inoculation experiments conducted by the mission at Camp Lazear (named for their esteemed compatriot), no fatal cases of yellow fever had occurred. Carroll was convinced of his ability to continue the experiments necessary to complete his work without unjustifiable risk to life. He proceeded to conduct the studies along the proposed plans and wrote Reed on August 22 to keep him informed of the plan to proceed with the filtration experiments.[6]

About a week later, Reed responded in a letter in which he reversed his views and advised Carroll to limit his observations to injection of serum alone without making controls injected with unfiltered blood. The following is an excerpt from Reed's letter to Carroll on August 27, 1901.

> I wrote you a few days ago advising against further experiments on human beings, in view of these fatal cases. From the tenor of your last letter, however, I see that you have made all preparations to go ahead with the observations as determined by us at Washington, and I hardly know what to say. I will suggest, that inasmuch as the injection of the blood has given us four positive results, you limit

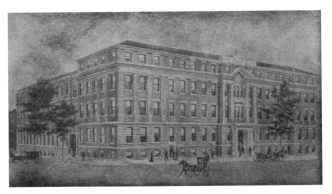

University Hospital, 1875

your observations to the injection of serum without making controls injected with unfiltered blood.[6]

Later after reflection, on August 29, 1901, Reed decided it unwise to interfere with Carroll's plans and cabled: "Consult Harvard. Use your own judgment in the future."

Carroll did complete his study and showed for the first time that the causative agent, present in the serum of yellow fever patients, was capable of passing through a filter which excluded bacteria, and that the agent in the blood was heat labile; heated blood from patients was noninfectious for volunteers. After Carroll completed his key work, on October 24, 1901, he answered a reprimand which he had received from the Army Adj. General of Cuba.

Howard Kelly, in his monograph on "Reed and Yellow Fever," says:

> All the reports of the Commission bear Doctor Carroll's name as well as that of Doctor Reed, and in reading them we should always bear in mind that, while the experiments were planned by the master mind of the chief, the accuracy with which they were carried out and the care by which all possible precautions were taken to exclude every source of error, are due to Doctor Carroll, quite as much as to Doctor Reed. (p. 266)[7]

William Welch, in reflecting upon Carroll's voluntary act of his illness and his conduct of the accurate and flawless experiments upon which the final conclusions of the Commission were based, remarked that Carroll was: "the most heroic of all the members," a comment which in no way was meant to detract

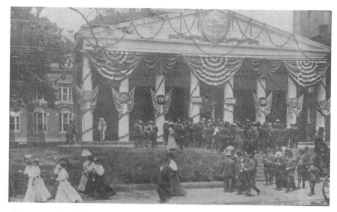

Centennial celebration at the University of Maryland School of Medicine, 1907

from the importance of the contributions and sacrifices made by other Commission members and volunteers.[8]

In the *British Medical Journal* of September 8, 1906, an editorial proposed that the Nobel Prize would be a "fitting acknowledgment of the work of these four men (Reed, Carroll, Lazear, Agramonte); it will scarcely be denied by anyone conversant with the facts."

General William C. Gorgas took his cue from the findings of the Reed Commission and conquered yellow fever first in Havana by isolation of yellow fever patients and eradication of *Aedes aegypti* mosquitoes. Such work made it possible to complete the Panama Canal which opened in 1914.

William T. Councilman, an 1878 University of Maryland graduate, and classmate of H.R. Carter, made a lasting contribution by describing the hepatic manifestations of yellow fever and description of a specific acidophilic body known universally as the "Councilman body," the hallmark of pathologic diagnosis.[9]

In 1976, various approaches to better treatment were evaluated in primates. Rhesus monkeys injected with the virulent ASIBI strain of yellow fever

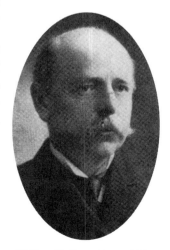

William T. Councilman, M.D.

virus, once infected, invariably died without treatment. After infection, survival time was significantly prolonged and several monkeys recovered fully following intravenous alimentation of concentrated nutritional fluids given via an indwelling catheter placed in the superior vena cava.

Another therapeutic approach conducted at USAMRIID (Frederick, Maryland) involved POLY ICCL (an interferon inducer). When given to monkeys 8 hours before injection of virulent ASIBI virus or 8 hours after infection occurred, the monkeys survived the infection—a unique accomplishment. Such use of intravenous alimentation or interferon had not been tested in humans.[6]

REFERENCES

1. Potter N. A Memoir of Contagion, More Especially as it Respects the Yellow Fever. Read at Convention of the Medical and Chirurgical Faculty of Maryland, June 1817. Published by Edward J. Coale, 1818.

2. Davidge JB. A Treatise on the Autumnal Endemial Epidemic of Tropical Climates, Commonly Called Yellow Fever, Containing its Origin, History, Nature and Cure, Together with a Few Reflections on the Proximate Cause of Disease. Printed by William Warner, 1813; first stated in 1798.

3. La Roche R. Yellow Fever Considered in Its Historical, Pathological, Etiological and Therapeutic Relations, Philadelphia, 1855.

4. Crawford J. A Lecture, Introductory to a Course of Lectures in the Cause, Seat and Cure of Diseases. Published by Edward J. Coale, 1811.

5. Carter HR. Note on interval between infecting and secondary cases of yellow fever from records at Orwood and Taylor, Miss. in 1898. New Orleans Med Surg J. 1900;52:617–638.

6. Woodward TE, Beisel WR, Faulkner RD. Marylanders defeat Philadelphia: Yellow fever updated. Trans Am Clin Climatol Assoc 1976;87:69–101.

7. Kelly, HA. Walter Reed and Yellow Fever. McClure Phillips and Company, 1906.

8. Welch WH. Address presented to the Johns Hopkins Historical Club Meeting, 14 October 1907. Held in memory of Major James Carroll, M.D., USA. Bull Johns Hopkins Hosp 1908;Jan:XIX.

9. Councilman WT. Pathologic histology of yellow fever. In Sternberg, G.M., ed. Report on Etiology and Prevention of Yellow Fever. U.S. Marine Hospital Service. Public Health Report: Bull No. 2, 151–159, 1980.

3

LEPROSY, MYCOTIC INFECTIONS, ACTINOMYCOSIS, AND SEXUALLY TRANSMITTED DISEASES

Theodore E. Woodward, M.D.

LEPROSY

Dr. George H. Rohe published his treatise on leprosy in 1878, the first report of this ancient disease in Maryland.[1] It included detailed reports of three cases observed for 10 years. He made significant contributions to the field of dermatology, particularly with respect to herpetic infections and venereal diseases.

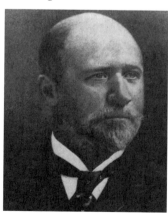

George H. Rohe, M.D.

Rohe graduated from the University of Maryland School of Medicine in 1873. He was Professor of Clinical Dermatology and Hygiene at the College of Physicians and Surgeons from 1878 to 1880. (It merged with the University of Maryland School of Medicine in 1915.)

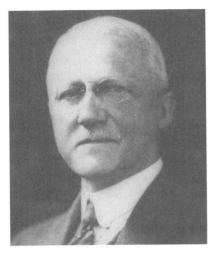

Thomas Gilchrist, M.D.

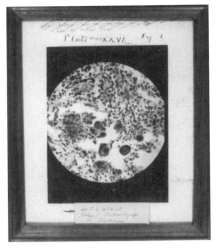

Photomicrograph of blastomycoses immitus (Gilchrist)

BLASTOMYCOSIS

Dr. Thomas Caspar Gilchrist described the first case of blastomycosis of the skin. His important contribution was the identification and isolation of the double-contoured spore, *Blastomyces dermatitidis*. Being a gifted artist, he made accurate drawings of the organisms as he viewed them under the microscope. These preparations are still valuable today.

Gilchrist, born on June 15, 1862, at Crewe, Cheshire, England, received his M.B. degree in London and came to America in 1889. After spending some time in Philadelphia, he entered practice in Baltimore. He was the first to hold the title of Clinical Professor of Dermatology at the Johns Hopkins Medical School in 1898, and simultaneously the position of Clinical Professor of Dermatology at the School of Medicine, University of Maryland, which he assumed in 1897. In 1907, Maryland awarded him the honorary degree of Doctor of Medicine.

HISTOPLASMOSIS

Dr. Samuel T. Darling (1903) made the initial report of a new disease, later identified as disseminated histoplasmosis, in Panama in 1906.[2] Darling predicted in his report in the *Journal of the Alumni Association of the College of Physicians, Baltimore* (January 1907, p. 102) that the "corresponding American disorder is

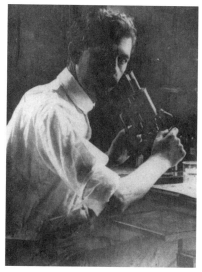

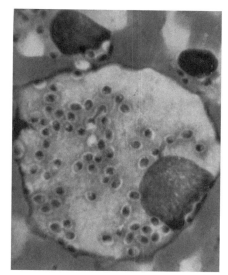

Samuel T. Darling, M.D.   *Stained smear of H. Capsulatum*

A PROTOZOÖN GENERAL INFECTION PRODUCING PSEUDOTUBERCLES IN THE LUNGS AND FOCAL NECROSES IN THE LIVER, SPLEEN AND LYMPHNODES.

SAMUEL T. DARLING, M.D.
Pathologist, Ancon Hospital.
ANCON, CANAL ZONE, ISTHMUS OF PANAMA.

On Dec. 7, 1905, while examining smears from the lungs, spleen and bone marrow in a case that appeared to be miliary tuberculosis of the lungs, I found enormous numbers of small bodies generally oval or round. Most of them were intracellular in alveolar epithelial cells, while others appeared to be free in the plasma of the spleen and rib marrow. Tubercle bacilli were absent.

FIGURE 3
Title and first paragraph of article first describing histoplasmosis. Reprinted with permission of the publishers of the J. A. M. A.

Title and first paragraph of article describing histoplasmosis.
(Reprinted with permission of the publishers of the JAMA.)

bound to appear in Baltimore some day. I hope it won't catch you napping."

Dr. Robert B. Wright, Professor of Pathology of the University of Maryland School of Medicine until his retirement in 1961, and Dr. Frank W. Hachtel, Professor and Chairman of the Department of Bacteriology from 1924 to 1954, were not caught unaware and reported the first documented case in Maryland. They identified the organism in tissues and isolated *Histoplasma capsulatum* from a fatal case, a diabetic bartender whose specific diagnosis was made before his death in March 1938.[3]

ACTINOMYCOSIS

Dr. John Rurah made the first collective investigation of actinomycosis in the United States, published in 1899–1900.[4] He graduated from the College of Physicians and Surgeons (later the University of Maryland) in 1894. He trained in Baltimore and abroad at the Pasteur Institute (Paris) and in Vienna and Berlin. In 1916, he became Professor of Pediatrics and Chairman of the Division, which was then a unit of the Department of Medicine.

His career was marked by distinction as a wise practitioner—learned, experienced, keen of insight, beloved, and honored as a cultured human being. He left a rich heritage of devoted service to medicine and humanity.

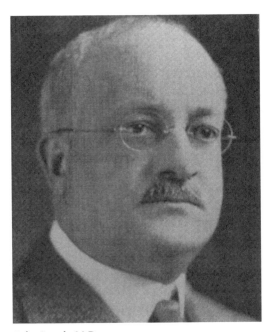

John Rurah, M.D.

GONORRHEA AND SYPHILIS

Newberry A.S. Keyser, while a student of medicine at the University of Maryland, published a convincing paper in 1883, which confirmed Neisser's observations of 1879 and 1882 that the gonococcus caused gonorrhea.[5] Also, he showed that Ehrlich's use of methylene blue as a stain, which he reported in 1881, was a reliable technique. This spread of bacteriologic knowledge and investigative evidence was remarkable, since Keyser, a medical student, provided information which antedated that of William Welch, a recognized authority in Baltimore and in the United States.

Keyser was born in 1860, went to Friends School and the Johns Hopkins University, and graduated from the University of Maryland School of Medicine in 1883. He remained in Baltimore until 1890, moved to Jerusalem, Harford County, and then moved to Upper Falls, Baltimore County, until 1929.

Beginning in 1948, Drs. Harry M. Robinson, Sr. and Harry M. Robinson, Jr., initiated studies of the efficacy of broad-spectrum antibiotics, such as chloramphenicol and Aureomycin and other tetracycline agents, in patients with the major venereal diseases.[6] These were the initial investigations which showed that gonorrhea and early syphilis could be effectively treated by oral

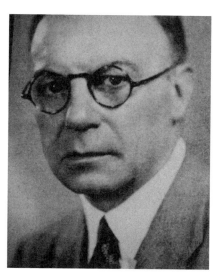

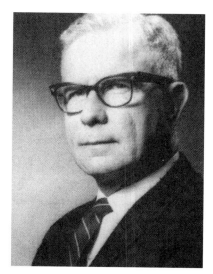

Harry M. Robinson, Sr., M.D.   *Harry M. Robinson, Jr., M.D.*

administration. At this point, the clinician had effective new forms of treatment when penicillin was ill-advised.

Robinson, Sr. greatly expanded the discipline of dermatology at the University of Maryland and developed it as a leading teaching center in the country.

Robinson, Jr. graduated in the Class of 1935. Following his house officership in medicine and special training in dermatology, he joined the faculty of medicine in 1941, served in the Armed Forces from 1941 to 1945, and was appointed Director of the Division of Dermatology in 1954 with the rank of full professor. He received numerous awards for his contributions to the field of dermatology and was Vice-President of the American Dermatological Association in 1975–1976.

REFERENCES

1. Rohe GH. Leprosy. Maryland Med J 1878;3:141–157.

2. Darling ST. A Protozoan general infection producing pseudo-tubercles in the lung and focal necrosis in the lever, spleen and lymph nodes. JAMA 1906;46:1283–1285.

3. Wright RB, Hachtel FW. Histoplasmosis of Darling: Report of a case. Ann Intern Med 1941;15:309.

4. Rurah J. Actinomycosis in man, with special reference to cases which have been observed in America. Ann Surg 1900;30:417–451, 31:235–241, 31:722–746.

5. Keyser NAS. Is gonorrhea a bacteria disease? Maryland Med J 1883;9:481–488.

6. Robinson HM Jr., Robinson HM Sr. Studies on chloramphenicol in early syphilis and gonorrhea. South Med J 1949;42:988–991.

4

RICKETTSIAL DISEASES

Theodore E. Woodward, M.D.

Interest in rickettsial diseases at University of Maryland is imbedded in its roots. The first systematic monograph of febrile illnesses in the United States was written by Elisha Bartlett, the second Professor of Theory and Practice of Medicine from 1844 to 1846.[1] His paper was the first worthwhile systematic discussion of typhus fever with minute and accurate analysis of signs and symptoms. His treatise on fevers was reproduced in four editions and immediately placed him in the front rank of American physicians of his time.

Much later, in 1930, two Maryland physicians identified the index case of murine typhus fever which led to the initial isolation of the causative Rickettsia from rats and fleas. In August 1930, a febrile patient, Dr. Joseph Lipsky, entered Mercy Hospital with high fever, prostration, headache, and general malaise. Lipsky had graduated from the College of Physicians and Surgeons, Baltimore in 1914. His physician, Louis A.M. Krause, and consultant, Maurice C. Pincoffs, made an initial diagnosis for typhoid fever, which was changed to typhus fever at the time of discharge, based on negative blood cultures and a positive proteus,

OX 19 reaction. These results were reported to authorities of the Public Health Service at the National Institutes of Health, Washington, D.C. Drs. Dyer, Rumreich, and Badger made an epidemiologic study of Lipsky's drugstore at Pennsylvania Avenue and Laurens Street. They identified a rickettsial agent in the brains of rats taken in the basement of the store and in fleas from the rodents. This was the index case of murine typhus fever (formerly called Brills' disease of endemic typhus fever) and opened a new concept of the ecology and reservoir of typhus fever.[2] Krause graduated from the University of Maryland with top honors in 1917.

The first report of an eastern variety of Rocky Mountain spotted fever (RMSF) came from Maryland in 1931.[3] One of three patients, reported by Dyer et al., was correctly identified by Maurice Pincoffs, who was familiar with the disease and who, as a medical student had contracted Colorado tick-bite fever while in the west. Today, it is known that RMSF is much more common in the east than in the west where it was first described by Ricketts in 1906.

During WWII in 1941, Capt. Theodore Woodward (Class of 1938), soon after his first overseas assignment in Jamaica,

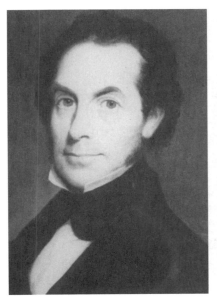

Elisha Bartlett, M.D.

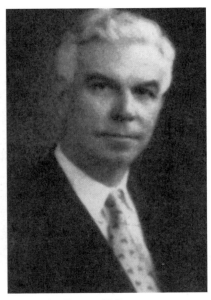

Louis A.M. Krause, M.D.

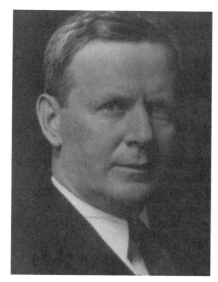

Maurice C. Pincoffs, M.D., M.A.C.P.

BWI, identified the first case of murine typhus fever on that island and in other Caribbean Islands.[4] The patient, a Jamaican laborer, developed a febrile illness with headache, prostration, myalgia, and continuous fever which masqueraded as malaria and failed to respond to quinine. The Weil-Felix test was positive. Confirmatory serologic studies were made at the Army Medical School, Army Medical Center, Washington, D.C. (WRAIR) where Woodward had trained. This identification of typhus fever stimulated further exploration of the rickettsial diseases in the Caribbean Islands and led to Woodward's further indoctrination in this field in Washington before going overseas.

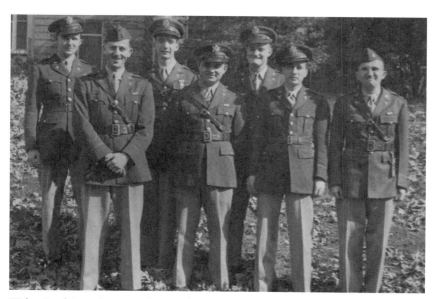

Walter Reed Army Institute of Research (WRAIR). Rear: Woodward, Hamilton, Philip. Front: Bukantz, Bennett, Bell, Reagan.

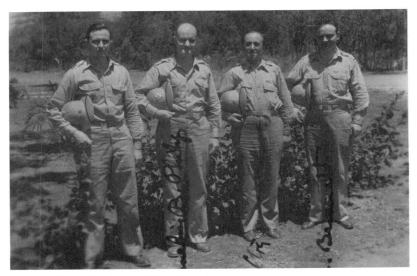

Jamaica, 1941: Woodward, Philip, Plotz, Bennett

Later, while working in North Africa at the Pasteur Institute, Morocco, as a member of the U.S.A. Typhus Fever Commission during World War (WW) II, Woodward conducted studies with French authorities in primates and in volunteers, which showed that one dose of an inactivated rickettsial typhus vaccine rapidly stimulated antibody formation and was protective against epidemic typhus.

EARLY USE OF VOLUNTEERS FOR EVALUATION OF VACCINE EFFICACY

Although not known at the time, this clinical vaccine trial was the forerunner of Maryland's program on vaccinology using human subjects. These seeds were planted in North Africa during the early stages of WW II (1943). Epidemic louse-borne typhus was endemic in Morocco, Algeria, and Tunisia and when the invasion occurred, typhus was present in epidemic proportions and posed a great threat to Allied military forces. American troops had been inoculated with an inactivated typhus vaccine, the efficacy of which was unknown. Woodward, assigned as a special medical officer to the Chief Surgeon NATOUSA, was subordinated for work on typhus based at the Pasteur Institute, Morocco. Through a serologic survey of American troops, he

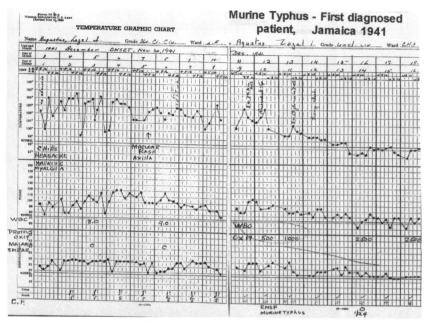

Murine typhus—first diagnosed patient, Jamaica, 1941

showed that they lacked serum antibodies, which could indicate susceptibility to infection. He then performed vaccine protection tests in guinea pigs and monkeys, and found that the presence of complement fixing antibodies at the time of injection of virulent typhus rickettsia indicated full protection against infection. His work was conducted in close collaboration with French health

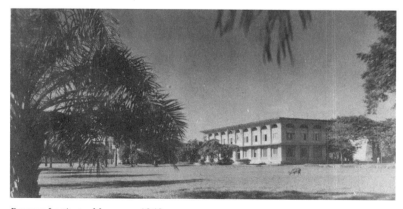

Pasteur Institute, Morocco, 1943

authorities, including the Secretary for Health Affairs. French and American authorities were most anxious to determine the best available vaccine and included a French product, which was untested. The American-type vaccine contained whole phenol-inactivated rickettsia. Top French and American authorities, including the U.S.A. Typhus Commission of which Dr. Woodward later became a member, agreed to a trial in volunteers. Healthy prison inmates, who freely volunteered as test subjects, were fully informed. Human controls were not employed because there was a clear threat of serious illness and possible death in the unvaccinated. The human trials conducted over a period of 18 months showed that the American-type vaccine afforded full protection after a virulent challenge of living R. prowazeki-type antibodies which were present in the serum at the time of challenge. Even one large dose instead of a three-dose weekly regimen was effective. After six months, those vaccinees, who had developed serum antibodies and then had become negative, developed only mild, almost asymptomatic, typhus after infection.

Hence, the stage was set with confidence that, if Allied military forces entered southern Europe or the Balkans in typhus-infested areas, such troops would be immune. Because of military security, these studies were not published until many years later.[5-7]

Tsutsugamushi disease or scrub typhus, as it became known, posed a new experience for Allied Forces in the southwest Pacific. It caused significant mortality and morbidity in troops who fought in northern Australia, New Guinea, and the various Pa-

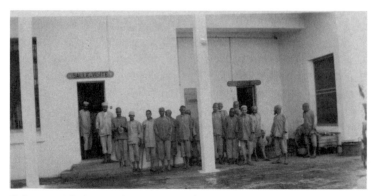

Volunteers (1943) in typhus vaccine trial

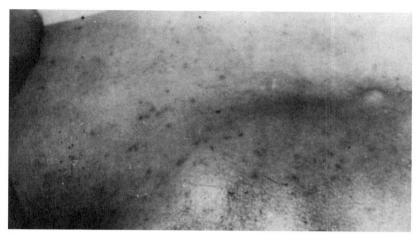

Epidemic typhus fever rash in volunteer

cific Islands as far as the Philippines. The U.S.A. Typhus Commission was active in developing new and necessary knowledge pertinent to prevention and treatment. Effective specific treatment came later. There were no available preventive vaccines, and the American troops lacked any immunity or resistance.

While working with Cornelius B. Philip, a leading entomologist, and others in 1944–1948, Maj. Woodward was able to localize new foci of the infection on Mindoro and Luzon where this serious rickettsial infection had never been identified. The same occurred for murine typhus, which was shown to be quite prevalent in rats in Manila, along with a few clinical cases.[8–11]

USE OF PABA IN RMSF

After WW II, interest in Rocky Mountain spotted fever greatly increased because of the availability of para-aminobenzoic acid (PABA), which had been reported to be of benefit in treatment. The availability of cases in Maryland made it possible to make extensive studies which showed very beneficial results, marked reduction in mortality, and shortening of the febrile course. The results of several large series of cases studied by Division members and house officers were reported. The only difficulty encountered was the rather troublesome side effects of the medication, particularly nausea and vomiting with occasional crystallization of PABA in the kidneys. Treatment was awkward and not well received by patients.

William (Bill) T. Raby, M.D., graduated in 1942, served with distinction in WW II in Europe, and completed his training in medicine at the University of Maryland, serving as Chief Medical Resident from 1947 to 1948. While at Maryland, he worked very actively in the patient treatment program which showed conclusively that para aminobenzoic acid was clinically beneficial.[12] He later settled in Charlotte, North Carolina and became a pillar of internal medicine there.

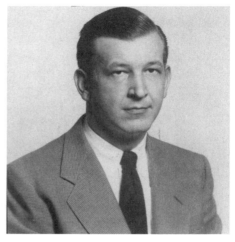

William T. Raby, M.D.

With this background of experience in rickettsial infection, the next series of events was the Typhus Medical Mission to Kuala Lumpur, Malaya, in 1948.

MEDICAL MISSION TO KUALA LUMPUR, MALAYA, IN 1948

After the war, scrub typhus fever remained an enigma; there was no vaccine and therapy with p-aminobenzoic acid was cumbersome. At the request of Dr. Joseph Smadel, Fred Stimpert, of Parke-Davis, provided him samples of any antimicrobial agents showing inhibitory properties for rickettsiae. Chloromycetin was included in a batch of possible candidates. With Betsy Jackson, this new streptomyces-derived antibiotic was shown to inhibit *Rickettsia orientalis* (scrub typhus) and lymphopathia venerium infections in fertile hens' eggs and mice. Joe Smadel and Herb Ley successfully treated a few cases of typhus in Mexico and demonstrated that blood levels of Chloromycetin occurred after oral administration.

During this period, Woodward migrated from Baltimore to WRAIR each Thursday to escape the rigors of clinical practice and exchange ideas about treatment of rickettsial diseases, including the use of PABA. Through authorities at WRAIR and the respective Departments of State, Smadel arranged the mission to Kuala Lumpur for testing the efficacy of Chloromycetin in scrub typhus. He selected the group: Herb Ley, scientific laboratory assistant to Smadel; Cornelius (Neil) Philip and Robert (Bob) Traub, entomologists; and Ted Woodward as clinician. The contract, (the first) funded at Maryland by the Medical Research and Development Command through the Commission on Immunization, of the AFEB, was awarded to the University of Maryland School of Medicine.

A special military transport plane carried the team and essential equipment. Raymond Lewthwaite, Director of the Institute for Medical Research, Kuala Lumpur, met the plane in Singapore on Sunday, March 14, 1948. The team immediately motored in jeeps through the green Malayan rain forest with its rubber plantations and isolated tin mines to the Selangor capital of Kuala Lumpur.

Dr. Lewthwaite took the team immediately to the bedside of a young Malayan soldier named Mohammed Osman, who had acquired his illness near the air strip in Kuala Lumpur. The history revealed headache, prostration, and fever of five days, and, upon examination, a tell-tale eschar from a mite-bite in the right axilla with adjacent adenopathy. After examination, blood was taken for the routine laboratory evaluation of hemoglobin, leukocyte count, acute-phase serum for the Weil-Felix reaction,

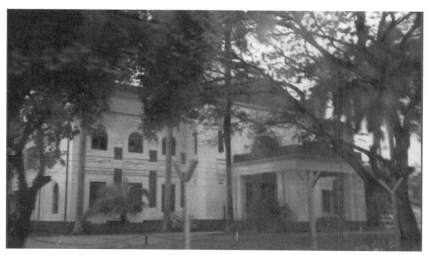

Institute for Medical Research, Kuala Lumpur, Malaya

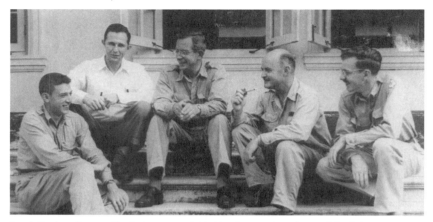

Scrub Typhus Group, Kuala Lumpur, 1948: Traub, Woodward, Smadel, Philip, Ley

and injection of mice intraperitoneally, for rickettsial isolation. A picture was taken of patient Osman in the hot mid-day sun. A loading oral dose of 2.0 g of Chloromycetin using 250-mg tablets was given with a subsequent schedule of one tablet every two hours until the 12th day of illness. Smadel had surmised that specific therapy should continue until emergence of proteus OX K agglutinins which usually occurred late in the second febrile week. By noon the next day, Osman was noticeably improved, less toxic in appearance, his headache was gone, and he

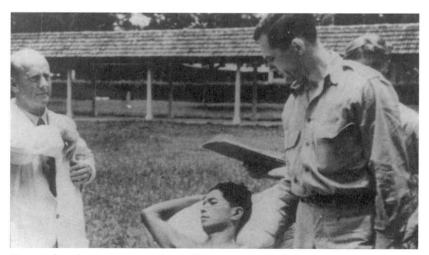

First scrub typhus patient treated with Chloromycetin, Kuala Lumpur, 1948

was afebrile 24 hours after beginning treatment. Subsequently, the diagnosis of scrub typhus was confirmed by isolation of Rickettsia and rise in titer of proteus OX K agglutinins. Recovery was prompt and complete without relapse.

The second patient was Corporal Bebbington of His Majesty's forces who was treated in the military hospital. Initially, quite ill, he responded promptly within 30 hours and did not relapse.

A steady flow of suspect typhus patients in the civilian and military hospitals of Kuala Lumpur, the nearby rubber estates, medical wards, and surrounding villages ensured an adequate clinical trial. Among these ill patients was a hardy group of Gurkha soldiers who were treated in the military hospital. There was no simultaneously untreated control series. Patients thought to have scrub typhus were selected and treated consecutively. Of the first 40 patients, 30 were confirmed as having scrub typhus. The additional 10 patients included two with murine typhus, two with malaria, one with blackwater fever, two with leptospirosis, two with typhoid (to be described later), and two with GKW (God knows what!). This represented a clinical diagnostic batting average of 75%.

The team experienced a striking example of the rapid spread of news. Lewthwaite received a telephone call from Stanley Pavillard, a prominent Singapore physician, whose patient, a banker, was desperately ill with typhus in its late stages. News reached Singapore via a British army officer traveling by train from Kuala Lumpur. Familiar with the recovery of Corporal Bebbington, he related the miraculous event to another passenger who was visiting the ill banker's family. Lewthwaite coerced Smadel, in spite of his protestations, to broaden the area of patient selection and send Woodward to treat the banker, Mr. Smith, in view of diplomatic amenities. The afternoon plane from Ipoh to Singapore was strewn with flowers and carried an urn containing a portion of the ashes of Mahatma Ghandi. Approximately 30,000 excited native Hindus met that plane. Pavillard cleverly extracted Woodward from the multitude and drove directly to the hospital. In spite of a domineering wife (a former nurse), and impending vascular collapse, delirium, and a purplish exanthem, Smith, case no. 9 in the series, recovered. This feat established beyond doubt that the antibiotic was remarkably effective at all stages.

Very early in the trials, Howard Florey (later Sir), then en route to London from Australia, stopped in Kuala Lumpur to observe the trials. After personally witnessing the 24-hour recovery of a scrub typhus patient and observing the clinical responses of the first few cases treated, which had been displayed graphically, Sir Howard remarked, "I'll buy it; you don't need statistical evidence."

Soon, it was clear that Chloromycetin cured scrub typhus patients promptly. Based on this confidence, the therapeutic regimen was reduced to one day's treatment and even one 3.0-g dose. All led to recovery without relapse, provided treatment was initiated not earlier than the fifth day of illness. Relapses were later encountered in patients treated prior to the fifth febrile day. These clinical results provided a basis for understanding the difficulties encountered in the subsequent chemoprophylactic field trials.

Initial Cure of Typhoid Fever

On Saturday night, April 3, 1948, the scrub typhus group was informed of two new febrile patients, numbers 17 and 18 in the initial series, who had been transported from a plantation that was ordinarily reliable as a source of scrub typhus patients. By candlelight, the brief clinical history and examination were completed, and specimens were obtained for laboratory evaluation. Both patients were toxic; neither had an eschar. Within 24 hours, one patient was improved dramatically in keeping with the prior experience. The second patient, number 18, was unchanged; he appeared toxic and apathetic, with abdominal distress and diarrhea. Enteric fever was suspected. Since blood cultures were not included in the routine, an attempt was made to retrieve typhoid bacilli from the peritoneal exudate of mice inoculated with blood. The smear was not confirmatory, but cultures of peritoneal exudate and other specimens of the patient's blood, yielded organisms. Therapy was continued. Smadel was annoyed that precious Chloromycetin tablets were being expended on a non-mission-oriented problem, but he relented. Within two days, some clinical improvement was apparent, based on bedside findings; defervescence occurred in about three days. Treatment was discontinued after five days of normal temperature; eight days later, the patient had a full-blown relapse and a toxic psychosis. The relapse responded to additional therapy.

The second selected typhoid patient responded in less than four days and did not relapse. Among the 10 treated typhoid patients, two relapsed, one became temporarily psychotic, another developed gross hemorrhage which required transfusion, and one experienced intestinal perforation with peritonitis and shock. All of the patients recovered. The group was convinced of the therapeutic benefit of Chloromycetin and published the results based on the 10 typhoid patients.[13]

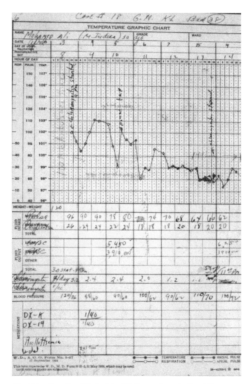

First patient with typhoid fever treated with Chloromycetin, 1948

Chemoprophylaxis of Scrub Typhus

After the obvious dramatic therapeutic response in scrub typhus patients, Joe Smadel directed the field prophylactic studies. American, English, and Malayan volunteers were purposely exposed by sitting eight hours daily for 10 days in a mite-ridden typhus-infested area.

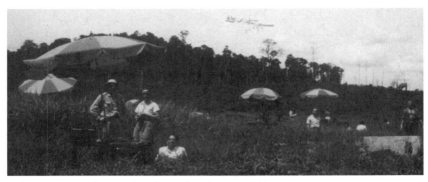

Volunteers exposed to scrub typhus-infected mites, 1948

Bob Traub, Cornelius Philip, and Ralph Audy had pin-pointed a highly infectious area at the Seaport Rubber Estate. These human field trials, which extended for several years, revealed that clinical typhus infection could be suppressed by administering the antibiotic at intervals once every four or five days for about seven weeks. Shorter, intermittent regimens resulted in rickettsemia and clinical illness. Giving Chloromycetin simultaneously, at the first day of infection, daily for 28 days, merely

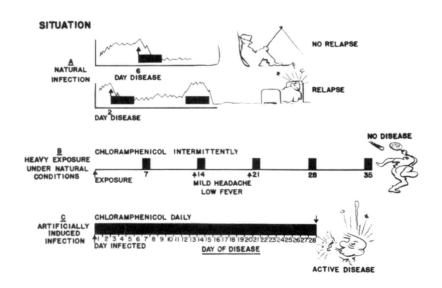

Relationship of chloramphenicol action and immunity in scrub typhus

extended the incubation period; classic illness occurred seven days after stopping the drug. The therapeutic findings in patients and results of the field trials in volunteers demonstrated the rickettsiostatic properties of Chloromycetin and established that resistance to infection bore a relationship to a sustained or sufficient intermittent antigenic stimulus. The field trials effectively demonstrated the immunologic relationships among host, microbe, and antibiotic and provided essential guidelines of chemoprophylaxis based on active immunization.[14–17] Charles Wisseman, Bennett Elisbert, Robert Traub, and others had a hand in these later studies. Smadel, himself a volunteer, developed a severe attack of typhus.

The initial venture to Kuala Lumpur ended in June 1948, with a total cost to the government of less than $50,000. This imaginative medical mission to Malaya was the forerunner of continued scientific collaboration between scientists of the IMR in Kuala Lumpur, WRAIR, and the University of Maryland. The new therapeutic, epidemiologic, and preventative techniques resulting from this international program are a fitting example of collaborative bi-national research.

STEROID TREATMENT OF TYPHOID FEVER

Fortified by knowledge that chloramphenicol effectively controlled the fever and acute manifestations of typhoid fever patients, the team directed attention to additional measures which might more rapidly ameliorate the toxic manifestations. Usually after initiating antibiotic treatment, toxic signs continued for about two days, and fever returned to normal levels in about three and one-half days. These were uniform findings. Studies by Maxwell Finland and others had shown that in pneumonia, corticosteroids favorably modified the toxic clinical signs, but that pneumococcal infection per se was enhanced by such treatment.

Shelly Greisman and his team of investigators, while evaluating the efficacy of typhoid vaccines in volunteers, showed that fever and toxic reactions of endotoxin (a lipopolysaccharide) could be modified in animals and humans and could actually be erased with corticosteroid administration (see Chapter 13).

Accordingly, chloramphenicol and a short-term cortisone regimen were used in typhoid patients in Baltimore and in Puerto Rico. Results were favorable. Toxic signs, including the fever, declined within 24 hours, and the results appeared excellent. Actually, several typhoid patients, treated in the later stages of illness, received cortisone solely with similar rapid abatement of toxicity and fever. Nevertheless, the team strongly recommended that combination specific antibiotic and steroids (used for several days only) be utilized in the severely ill and not routinely. Similar findings using steroids were observed in Rocky Mountain spotted fever, brucellosis, and tularemia (described in other chapters). Various clinicians who treated typhoid patients with corticosteroids noted favorable results without untoward effects using short-term regimens. However, the point was never proven or confirmed by a statistically controlled study.[18]

In 1981, Navy Lieutenant Stephen Hoffman, while serving on assignment in Jakarta, Indonesia, wrote comprehensively that in his area and in other known foci of typhoid fever, deaths occurred from typhoid in spite of specific antibiotic treatment. It was suggested to him that a controlled study of corticosteroids and specific antibiotic treatment be performed on a controlled basis, provided there were sufficient numbers of patients. He initiated a controlled study involving seriously ill patients either in shock or impending shock. Clear-cut criteria were established. One group received chloramphenicol alone and another received combinations of chloramphenicol and high-dose dexamethasone for three days. Greisman helped plan the dosage of dexamethasone based on a mg/kg basis. After initiating the study, Hoffman's group noticed that after studying about 20 patients, there was a distinct difference in response. Although they were unfamiliar with the treatment code (antibiotic vs. antibiotic/steroid group), they surmised, based on clinical judgment, that the results differed significantly and presumed that the few fatal cases were in the antibiotic group. It was then arranged for a British infectious disease authority from Singapore to visit Jakarta and examine the data. After his evaluation, he strongly recommended stopping the study because the few deaths which occurred were in the group given antibiotic alone. Ethically, there was no other decision.[19-21] The study was continued using double therapy solely with antibiotic and steroids. The results were convincingly favorable for the benefit of steroids in severely ill/toxic typhoid patients. The public is indebted to the Department of the Navy and U.S. Department of Defense for this landmark contribution.

Later, Dr. Wesley Spink of the University of Minnesota called to gratefully acknowledge the suggestion and inform us that cortisone successfully abated the toxic manifestations of the Jarisch-Herxheimer reaction in antibiotic-treated patients with acute brucellosis.

REFERENCES

1. Bartlett E. The History, Diagnosis and Treatment of Typhoid and Typhus Fever. Lea and Blanchard: Philadelphia 1842.

2. Dyer RE, Rumreich AS, Badger LF. The typhus-Rocky Mountain spotted fever group in the United States. JAMA 1931;97:589–595.

3. Dyer RE, Rumreich AS, Badger LF, Pincoffs MC, Shaw CC. The eastern type of Rocky Mountain spotted fever. Report of a case with demonstration of Rickettsia. Med Clin North Am 1933; 16:1097–1113.

4. Plotz H, Woodward TE, Philip CB, Bennett BL, Evans KL. Endemic typhus fever in Jamaica, B.W.I. Am J Public Health 1943;33: 812–814.

5. Official report to Chief Surgeon, NATOUSA, Director USA Typhus Fever Commission and Chief Preventive Medicine Section, Office of the Surgeon General (Army) December 1942. History of Preventive Medicine in World War II, Office of the Surgeon General, Department of the Army, 1964.

6. Woodward TE. Murine and epidemic typhus rickettsia: How close is their relationship? Yale J Biol Med 1982;55:335–341.

7. Woodward TE. Rickettsial vaccines with emphasis on epidemic typhus: Initial report of an old vaccine trial. South African Med J 1986; Oct. 11:73–76.

8. Philip CB, Woodward TE. Two new species of rat mites (Neoschongastiaspp) from a focus of scrub typhus in Mindoro, Philippine Islands. Am J Trop Med 1946;26:157–163.

9. Philip CB, Woodward TE, Sullivan, RR. Tsutsugamushi disease (scrub or mite-borne typhus) in the Philippine Islands during the American reoccupation in 1944–1945. Am J Trop Med 1946;26:229–242.

10. Woodward TE, Philip CB, Loranger GL. Endemic typhus in Manila, Philippine Islands. Report of cases and identification of the murine rickettsial agent in domestic rats by complement fixation. J Infect Dis 1946;78:167–172.

11. Philip CB, Woodward TE. Tsutsugamushi disease (scrub or mite-borne typhus) in the Philippine Islands during the American reoccupation in 1944–45. II. Observations on Trombiculid. J Parasitol 1946;32: 504–513.

12. Woodward TE, Raby WT. Further concepts in the treatment of Rocky Mountain spotted fever with para-aminobenzoic acid. South Med J 1948;41:997–1003.

13. Woodward TE, Smadel JE, Ley HL Jr, Green R, Mankikar DS. Preliminary report on the beneficial effect of Chloromycetin in the treatment of typhoid fever. Ann Intern Med 1948;29:131–134.

14. Woodward TE, Smadel JE, Ley HL Jr, Green R, Mankikar DS. Preliminary report on the beneficial effect of Chloromycetin in the treatment of typhoid fever. Ann Intern Med 1948;29:131–134.

15. Smadel JE, Woodward TE, Ley HL Jr, Philip CB, Traub R, Lewthwaite R, Savoor SR. Chloromycetin in the treatment of scrub typhus. Science 1948;108:160–161.

16. Smadel JE, Woodward TE, Ley HL Jr, Lewthwaite R. Chloramphenicol (Chloromycetin) in the treatment of tsutsugamushi disease (scrub typhus). J Clin Invest 1949;28:1196–1215.

17. Smadel JE, Traub R, Ley, HL Jr, Philip CB, Woodward TE, Lewthwaite R. Chloramphenicol (Chloromycetin) in the chemoprophylaxis of scrub typhus (tsutsugamushi disease). II. Results with volunteers exposed in hyperendemic areas of scrub typhus. Am J Hyg 1949;50: 75–91.

18. Woodward TE, Hall HE, Parker RT. Cortisone as an ancillary aid in the treatment of typhoid fever. Trans Am Clin Climatol Assoc 1950;62:1.

19. Smadel JE, Ley HL Jr, Diercks FH. Treatment of typhoid fever. I. Combined therapy with cortisone and chloramphenicol. Ann Intern Med 1951;34:1–9.

20. Woodward TE, Hall HE, Dias-Rivera R, Hightower JA, Martinez E, Parker RT. Treatment of typhoid fever II, control of clinical manifestations with cortisone. Ann Intern Med 1951;1(Jan):10–19.

21. Hoffman SL, Punjabi NH, Kumala S, Moechtar MA, Pulungsih SP, Rival AR, Rockhill RC, Woodward TE, Loedin AL. Reduction of mortality in chloramphenicol-treated severe typhoid fever by high-dose dexamethasone. N Engl J Med 1984;310(Jan):82–88.

5

BEGINNINGS, ORGANIZATION, AND EARLY ACTIVITIES OF THE DIVISION OF INFECTIOUS DISEASES

Theodore E. Woodward, M.D.

BACKGROUND AND BEGINNING

Prior to World War II, medical schools seldom sponsored research, educational, or practice programs dealing *specifically* with infectious diseases. New information in this field, including problems dealing with applied epidemiology, came from institutions especially versed along these lines. These included the Division of Biological Standards of the NIH, the Rockefeller and Thorndike and Evans Memorial Centers, the Walter Reed Army Institute for Research, Schools of Public Health and Hygiene (such as at Harvard, Johns Hopkins, Michigan, Pittsburgh, Louisiana, the Hooper Foundation, San Francisco), Departments of Microbiology or Epidemiology in medical schools, the Biologic Division at Johns Hopkins, special schools in tropical and international medicine (such as at London and Hamburg), and the systems of Pasteur Institutes, which were all in the forefront. Faculty members in veterinary or medical schools made important contributions.

World War II witnessed much focus on infectious disorders, particularly malaria, hepatitis, and respiratory, enteric, rickettsial, and wound infections which took heavy tolls. Specialization began with an explosion after the war and soon infectious diseases units developed in medical schools widely throughout the United States.

EARLY DEVELOPMENT OF
INFECTIOUS DISEASES PROGRAM AT MARYLAND

After World War II, Woodward entered medical practice sharing an office with Samuel T.R. Revell and Edward F. Cotter at 11 E. Chase Street, Baltimore. They taught at the Medical School and Hospital and conducted clinical research on a volunteer basis while engaged in private medical practice. Every Thursday afternoon, Woodward went to the Walter Reed Army Research Center in order to work at the old Rickettsial Disease Laboratory, where Joe Smadel had settled as Scientific Director. Work continued on murine typhus and

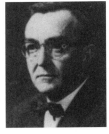

Samuel T.R. Revell, Jr., M.D.

spotted fever since para-aminobenzoic acid had come into vogue as treatment. Spring and summer found the small group busy examining cases with Rocky Mountain spotted fever (RMSF) in various Baltimore hospitals and throughout the state. Many Maryland patients were referred to the University Hospital. Laboratory work with blood specimens and guinea pigs was performed on open laboratory table counters begin-

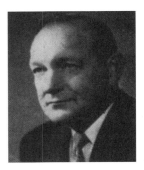

Edward F. Cotter, M.D.

ning in the Bacteriology Laboratory of the Basic Science Building. Dr. Frank Hachtel, Chairman of Bacteriology, had kindly made laboratory space available and only later was it possible to obtain facilities on the fifth floor of the Bressler Building. In reflecting back, it was fortunate that cross-infection of RMSF did not occur, since the facilities were primitive and dangerous. There was no protective hood. Dr. Perrin Long had invited Woodward to teach Preventive Medicine at the Hopkins School of Public Health and Hygiene. There were restrictions there against handling pathogenic agents, such as rickettsia, which precluded performing this research activity at Hopkins.

The Thursday afternoons at Walter Reed, added to the other times spent there, at odd hours, solidified an even closer relationship with Joe Smadel and the talented staff of that fine research institute. These weekly experiences really afforded Woodward much needed postgraduate laboratory experience in continuing scientific education. Actually, at that time, there were no rickettsiologists in Baltimore with whom to share the intellectual stimulation so sorely needed. In this setting, at Walter Reed, the new antibiotic Chloromycetin, identified and produced by Parke-Davis, Detroit, was to undergo its early clinical evaluation. In 1948, an opportunity arose which probably had significant far-reaching influence on Maryland's research programs.

What followed was the typhus medical mission to Kuala Lumpur, Malaysia, in 1948 (described in Chapter 4). There, we were fortunate enough to find the first cure for scrub, murine typhus fever, and typhoid fever and evolve an interrupted antibiotic regimen to prevent scrub typhus in volunteers.

One evening, later in 1948, after the successful scientific venture to Kuala Lumpar, Dr. and Mrs. Maurice C. Pincoffs graciously entertained Woodward and his wife Celeste for dinner at their lovely home, Markland, along Old Frederick Road. After dinner, in the living room, Dr. Pincoffs did not press an offer, but in his careful and wise way indicated that a full-time position at Maryland was advisable. He stated that Maryland needed to develop medical resident training programs and research. The offer was enthusiastically accepted.

Up to 1948, there were no full-time teachers in clinical medicine or in any other disciplines at the University of Maryland School of Medicine and Hospital. Maurice Pincoffs was paid a small part-time salary as Chairman of the Department of Medicine. The only partially structured specialty divisions in the department were Cardiology, under Dr. William S. Love; Physical Diagnosis, under Dr. Conrad Wolff; Dermatology, directed by Dr. Harry M. Robinson, Sr.; and Clinical Pathology, under Dr. John Huck. Dr. Milton Sacks, then at the Mercy Hospital, joined the Department as Head of Clinical Pathology in 1947, which included Hematology. The total legislative budget of the Department of Medicine was less than $50,000 per annum, which included secretarial assistance and small payments to various practitioners/teachers.

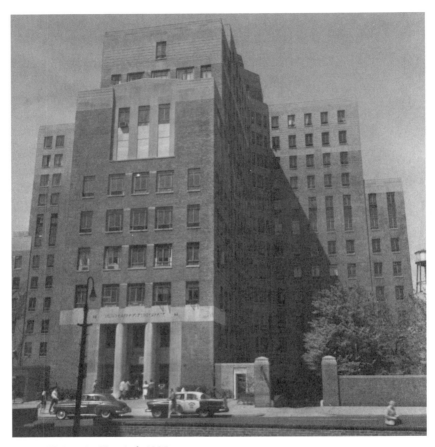

"New" University Hospital, 1935

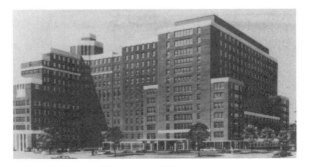

University Hospital Complex, 1981

Woodward joined the department as the first *geographical* full-time Professor–Department of Medicine, with limited practice privilege. Most of the teaching of medical students and a small house staff, as well as patient care, was rendered by dedicated and very effective part-time nonsalaried physicians who were engaged in active medical practice in Baltimore and surrounding areas.

FORMAL INITIATION OF INFECTIOUS DISEASES PROGRAM

Beginning in 1948, new specialty divisions in medicine were organized and developed with an active teaching and research program initiated in infectious diseases which Woodward directed from 1948 to 1954. This was one of the first specifically named divisions in a department of medicine, along with Hopkins and Cornell.

Merrill J. Snyder, a protégé of Col. Harry Plotz and Joseph E. Smadel of the Rickettsial Diseases Laboratory at the Army Medical School (later WRAIR), was recruited from Washington to

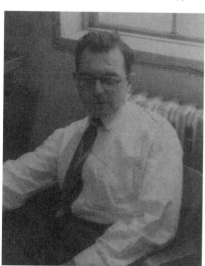

Merrill J. Snyder, Ph.D.

Baltimore in 1949, to assist in the development of the new and growing division. His expert competence in serology and microbiological techniques was most helpful and essential. Merrill had broad professional capability and was most effective in teaching medical students, house officers, and fellows. He served as the Division's Socrates in terms of collection and interpretation of valid statistical data. Ann Meredith was the first technician who participated in all activities and was a great help. She contracted tularemia from pipetting infected material, but quickly recovered with treatment. By this time, we had acquired laboratory space on the fifth floor of the Bressler Building which had been kindly made available by Dr. J. Mason Hundley,

Chairman of OB/GYN. Animal inoculation was frequently used at the time, which created a contaminated environment because of limited facilities. From 1948 to 1950, assistant residents in medicine spent time as fellows in the new research unit. Leonard Lister, a medical resident, also developed tularemia and pneumonia through pipetting solutions from a test tube culture. Chloramphenicol quickly cured him. Soon we were able to acquire a hooded protective unit which helped greatly.

The first division secretary was Audrey Taylor who came when Woodward left private medical practice in late 1948. She was soon followed by Martha Carol Young. Mrs. Young was most precise, disciplined, and ran a tight ship, which was very fortunate, indeed, because of the growing responsibilities and ultimate need to administer large grants-in-aid from various government agencies. Later these included the NIH and the USA Research and Development Command of the Department of Defense, as well as pharmaceutical companies. All of these had to be administered through a very tight fiscal network headquartered at College Park. Later in 1954, Mrs. Young became the head secretary of the Department of Medicine when Woodward assumed the post of Department Chairman.

In the early period, virulent microorganisms were handled, such as those causing RMSF, epidemic typhus fever, murine typhus fever, scrub typhus fever, and Q-fever. Brucellae and

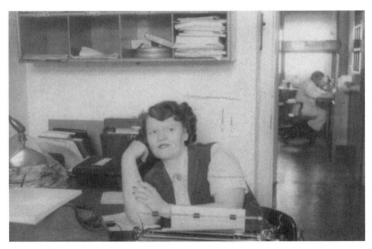

M. Carol Young, Department Administrator

tularemia were injected into animals, and postmortem tissues were examined on open counters. Culture techniques were performed under these very limited facilities. There were no hoods or normal protective devices. Media had to be made, and glassware was cleaned by hand and sterilized individually. Fortunately, there were no serious mishaps.

This initial unit, and the larger one to follow, served as a special diagnostic service for the hospital and interested groups requesting such support services. There were no charges for the services. Serologic procedures including agglutination tests, were performed for everyone for brucellosis, tularemia, and complement fixation reactions for the rickettsial diseases and certain viruses such as lymphocytic choriomeningitis (LCM), lymphopathia venerium (LGV), and some others. Residents and fellows helped in performing this work.

The initial grant in 1948, in the amount of $10,000, came from the McCormick Spice Company, Inc., through the generosity of its president, Charles P. McCormick, Sr. This made it possible to pursue studies on the efficacy of antibiotics, particularly Chloromycetin and tetracycline. These studies were performed in Baltimore and Puerto Rico where we established excellent working relationships. The McCormick Fund made this possible. Serious infectious diseases, such as typhoid fever, RMSF, meningitis, brucellosis, tularemia, bacteremia, and plague, were investigated intensively in Baltimore and abroad. The McCormick Company made second and third awards in the following years which allowed us to organize on a

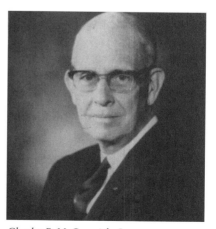

Charles P. McCormick, Sr.

more solid base and expand the research center in Puerto Rico where our interest and capabilities in infectious diseases expanded. A generous gift came from Parke-Davis, Detroit; their full support extended over several decades. These developments allowed the division to expand, to purchase essential equipment, recruit new personnel, and initiate a formalized fellowship program. Dr. William Holbrook, who became a top surgeon, was the first fellow.

Additional awards soon came from other pharmaceutical firms such as the Lederle Laboratories, Pfizer, and Wyeth & Company. With these beginnings, and favorable progress, support followed from the various federal agencies, as previously mentioned.

Getting started on a new research program is a problem for any new and inexperienced group. Parke-Davis alone, beginning in 1952 and up to 1975, contributed approximately $250,000 annually for support of mutually beneficial programs on antimicrobial use and basic medical research. This was a prime example of meaningful collaboration between a pharmaceutical company and an academic center.

During this active period, 1948–1952, Woodward served as a member of the Commissions on Rickettsial Disease and Epidemiological Survey of the Armed Forces Epidemiological Board (AFEB). He was a member of the Commission of Epidemiological Survey from 1952 to 1959 and its Chairman from 1959 to 1973. Dr. Richard Shope, a distinguished biologist at the Rockefeller Institute, was the first Chairman and served from 1952 to 1959. This program, centered at Fort Detrich, Maryland, was directly charged by our government for developing knowledge about defense against biological warfare. The activities of the Division of Infectious Disease fitted in nicely with the objectives of the Commission of Epidemiologic Survey and were directly responsible and accountable for the growth and the maturity of the division. The program now involved research of new knowledge dealing with the pathogenesis and control of serious pathogenic infections (i.e., plague, typhus, typhoid, dysentery, Q fever, tularemia, brucellosis, Rift valley fever, and others). Actually, a symbiotic relationship developed between the two centers which was essential for development of new knowledge in these fields. These activities were directly related to the expansion of the human vaccine testing program.

USE OF VOLUNTEERS

The very first use of volunteers at Maryland involved the study of typhoid fever. The successful demonstration, in 1948, that

Chloromycetin successfully cured patients with typhoid vaccine made it possible to access the efficacy of typhoid vaccine in humans. There were no reliable animals to use except the chimpanzee, whose response to the disease closely imitated the reaction in humans, but the illness in chimps was not fully comparable. During a session of the AFEB at WRAIR, Col. Hershall Griffin, MC, Chief Preventive Medical Officer, stated that in Europe, a vaccine tablet containing inactivated typhoid bacilli was widely used to prevent typhoid fever. Its value was under question. Woodward asked the Board if it wished to have the vaccine efficacy tested in humans. A committee was appointed by Dr. Gustave (Gus) Dammin to address the problem. The ability to control the illness in volunteers, without serious hazard, made such testing feasible. The AFEB approved the proposal in 1950. Woodward then posed the question to Dr. Pincoffs, his Chief, Dean Wylie of the Medical School, President H.C. Byrd, and the Board of Regents of the University of Maryland. There were no peer review committees at that time. All persons were fully informed of the various considerations involved. Approval was given to proceed. At that time, there were two Maryland penitentiary trustee inmates on the medical wards with minor illness unrelated to typhoid fever. They were fully informed of the various considerations and potential developments. They freely volunteered without compensation. The two current medical advisors for the penal system in Maryland were Dr. John T.

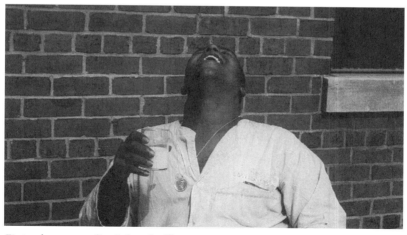

First volunteer gargling infected milk

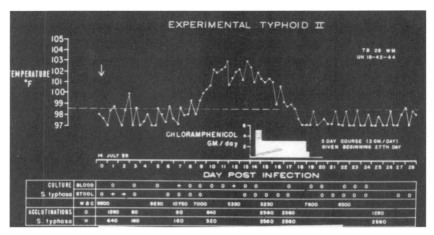

Typical clinical course of volunteer with typhoid fever

King and Dr. Henry L. Thomas, senior and respected physicians in Maryland. They were consulted for advice and gave their full consent for the testing.

After full consent by the two volunteers, their examination consisted of complete assessment of their general health, including negative findings regarding a prior typhoid infection (they all tested negative). An attempt was being made, as the first step, to determine the infectious dose of typhoid bacteria necessary to infect a human. There were no available data from the current literature. The inoculum was prepared at WRAIR by Dr. Joseph Smadel and Dr. Robert Traub using the old Ty2 strain. It was originally isolated from a soldier who developed typhoid fever in Cuba during the Spanish American War (1898). For many years, this strain had been transferred repeatedly in test tube cultures to maintain its viability. We had decided initially to use 600 whole living typhoid bacilli as the first attempt. The infectious inoculum was placed in milk. The volunteers were instructed to gargle the emulsion, in order to infect the tonsillar area, and then swallow it. This was done after breakfast with the thought that food in the stomach would neutralize the gastric acid and make infection more likely.

All types of follow-up studies were performed several times daily and included cultures of the pharynx, gastric content, stool, blood, and bone marrow. Also the appropriate serologic test (i.e., the Widal typhoid agglutination reaction) was performed.

Joe Smadel and Bob Traub came from WRAIR to deliver the infectious cocktail and witness its administration. On returning to Washington, Bob Traub called, somewhat excitedly, and said, "we missed a decimal point, there were 6,000 not 600 typhoid bacilli." However, nothing happened!—no fever, no clinical signs of typhoid, and *all* cultures were negative. There was no evidence of serologic conversion. This experience taught us a lesson: results in the test tube, mouse, or monkey are not always comparable to results in man. They differ, and one cannot extrapolate one from the other. Later, Dr. Thomas Francis, who had studied hepatitis virus infections in prison volunteers in Michigan, remarked to Woodward at an AFEB meeting, "Ted, you had better use a recently humanized strain of typhoid bacilli." The old Ty2 stain had lived in a test tube for about 50 years.

We then obtained a strain of fresh bacilli from Mrs. Lillie Quailes, a typhoid carrier from the Eastern Shore of Maryland whom we had previously treated. Her typhoid strain had infected several members of her family, some rather severely. We had noted that her bile contained approximately 60,000,000 typhoid bacilli per ml of bile. This strain became the standard one which we used for all of our subsequent studies of typhoid vaccines in volunteers which will be described later.

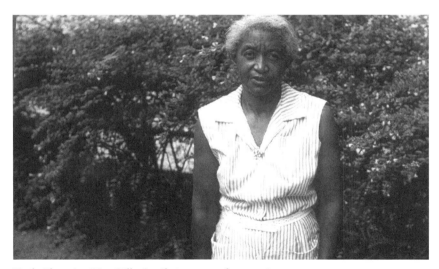

Typhoid carrier (Mrs. Lilly Quailes), source of test strain

PERSONNEL CHANGES

Dr. Robert T. Parker, a former fellow in infectious diseases, continued the division's activities as an effective teaching, research, and consulting service on the campus, and succeeded Woodward who had served from 1948 to 1954 as director of the division. Parker chaired the division until 1957. Dr. Fred R. McCrumb, Jr. joined in the early investigative work and directed the division from 1957 to 1963. McCrumb's contribution to our knowledge of leptospirosis and measles vaccine is of lasting importance. He, because of his leadership capabilities, was appointed director of the school's program in tropical medicine and international health training in the new research center in Lahore, West Pakistan. Dr. Richard B. Hornick, a graduate of the Johns Hopkins School of Medicine, joined the department after military service at Fort Detrick. While there, he was actively involved in the Tularemia Program with Col. Ed Overholt and others with whom the division associated. Hornick brought a keen clinical and research sense and served first as chief medical resident. He became director of the division in 1963. Under his leadership, which continued until 1979, clinical studies on the pathogenesis, prevention, and control of infectious diseases were expanded. The volunteer program became a model of its type and during the next several decades, with support from the World Health Organization (WHO), it contributed much new knowledge on pathogenesis, treatment, prevention, and control with further use of vaccines. Dr. Stephen C. Schimpff, Head of the Division of Infectious Diseases of the Baltimore Cancer Research Program, succeeded Hornick as Head of the Division of Infectious Diseases in 1979. In addition to his clinical skills, Schimpff made important contributions regarding infections in patients with malignant disorders under immunosuppression. He served as Division Head until 1983. During the gaps when there was change of division leadership, Merrill Snyder often served as a most effective interim director.

From July 1984 until September 1985, Michael (Mike) Levine was Acting Head of the Division of Infectious Diseases. Mike graduated from the Medical College of Virginia in 1967 and from 1970 to 1972 was a fellow in the division, then headed by Richard Hornick. Levine was an assistant professor of medicine, then an associate professor from 1975 to 1981, and finally a

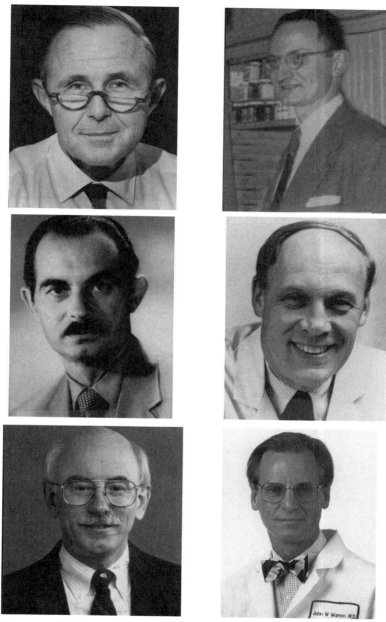

Directors of the Division of Infectious Diseases: (Top row) Theodore E. Woodward, M.D. (1948–1954); Robert T. Parker, M.D. (1954–1957); (Middle row) Fred R. McCrumb, Jr., M.D. (1957–1963); Richard B. Hornick, M.D. (1963–1979); (Bottom row) Stephen C. Schimpff, M.D. (1979–1983); John W. Warren, M.D. (1986–present)

full professor in 1982. His research contributions in the field of vaccinology have been prodigious. In 1974, he was made responsible for the program in vaccine development which was officially designated a Center in 1983. He became Head of the Division of Geographic Medicine of the department in 1984.

Dr. John (Jack) Warren, a Harvard graduate, class of 1970, served his house-officership at Case Western Reserve, a fellowship in infectious diseases from 1974 to 1976 at Harvard, and was appointed to our faculty as Assistant Professor of Medicine in Infectious Diseases in 1977. His interests have embraced upper and lower urinary tract infections and their means of control. Warren was appointed Head of the Division in 1986 and promoted to the rank of Professor in 1990.

Fred McCrumb recruited Ann S. Schluderburg, S.C.D., from the virology section of the Hopkins School of Public Health as a junior faculty member in the division in 1959. She contributed importantly to the studies which confirmed the efficacy of measles virus vaccine in children (1962). Her work on immune globulin was a significant contribution. Drs. McCrumb and Hornick were her colleagues. Schluderburg then transferred to Yale and in 1979 moved to the NIAID, NIH in Bethesda, Maryland.

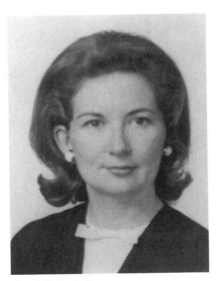

Ann S. Schluderburg

6

CONTINUATION OF STUDIES ON RICKETTSIOSIS

Theodore E. Woodward, M.D.

FIRST SPECIFIC CURE OF ROCKY MOUNTAIN SPOTTED FEVER

While the antibiotic efficacy studies were being performed in Malaya, Dr. Maurice Pincoffs and a small group of physicians made similar clinical observations at the University Hospital.[1] A small supply of Chloromycetin had been given to Dr. Pincoffs for testing in patients with Rocky Mountain spotted fever (RMSF) contracted in Maryland. The results were dramatic, and treatment led to prompt and favorable response. Hence a serious and commonly fatal illness came under control. (For information on identification, transmission, and vaccine for RMSF, see "Rocky Mountain Spotted Fever" section later in this chapter.)

PATHOPHYSIOLOGICAL ALTERATIONS IN SEVERE RICKETTSIOSES

One of the important clinical observations made regarding the pathophysiologic abnormalities in a major rickettsiosis, epidemic typhus fever, involved the status of the circulatory system. Standard concepts in 1940 dictated that the central circulation and the heart accounted for the vascular instability and weakness. The avoidance of intravenous fluids and use of digitalis even in the early stages of illness were stressed in standard texts with respect to treatment of patients with typhus and RMSF. In North Africa, working in collaboration with Dr. Edward Bland and Dr. Daniel Ellis of the 6th General Hospital (Massachusetts General Hospital), it was shown that just the reverse was true; venous pressures were low rather than high, the vascular collapse was related to low blood volume associated with hyponatremia, and intravenous fluids were not only useful, but occasionally needed at that early stage of illness. Only in the later stages of illness, at the height of the vascular pathologic changes and increase in capillary permeability, was it necessary to restrict fluids. When our studies on typhus fever in North Africa were made and published,[2] Dr. George Harrell reported similar findings in patients with RMSF studied in North Carolina.

INITIAL REPORT OF ANTITOXEMIC EFFECTS OF CORTICOSTEROIDS ON PATIENTS WITH TYPHOID FEVER AND ROCKY MOUNTAIN SPOTTED FEVER

Various staff members of the Department of Medicine of the University of Maryland School of Medicine and Hospital reported the results of clinical trials of the efficacy of corticosteroids in patients seriously ill with typhoid fever (1950) and Rocky Mountain spotted fever (1951). Dramatic reduction in toxic signs of illness and rapid defervescence occurred usually within 24 hours of initiating steroid treatment in conjunction with antibiotics. These investigators concluded that corticosteroids were therapeutically indicated only in those patients seriously ill with these diseases who were encountered late in illness, and that broad-spectrum antibiotics remained the mainstays of management.[3]

EARLY FUNDAMENTAL STUDIES OF PATHOGENESIS AND PHYSIOLOGIC ABNORMALITIES IN RICKETTSIAL DISEASES

Beginning in 1951, Dr. Charles L. Wisseman, Jr. and his associates made the initial report of a series of fundamental studies designed to clarify the pathogenesis and physiologic abnormalities in various rickettsial diseases, specifically the typhus fevers and Rocky Mountain spotted fever, as a guide to developing a better

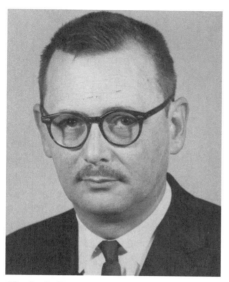

Charles L. Wisseman, Jr., M.D.

means of diagnosis, prevention, and management.

Particularly significant was the initial elucidation of the composition of rickettsiae[4] and the fundamental investigations on the mechanisms of action of rickettsial toxins.[5] The later work of Wisseman clarified the chemotactic and phagocytic events following introduction of rickettsiae into the host.[6]

After graduation from the Southwestern Medical School, Wisseman was a house officer in medicine. He received specialized training in parasitology and joined the United States Army with assignment at the Army Medical Service Graduate School in 1948, where he initiated his rickettsial studies. In 1954, Wisseman was appointed Professor and Chairman of the Department of Microbiology at the University of Maryland School of Medicine. He continued his basic work and developed a strong program for teaching medical and graduate students.

Bob Traub contributed most importantly to our knowledge of rickettsial diseases. Without doubt, he was one of our nation's leading entomologists. He joined the Maryland Faculty in the Department of Microbiology, under Dr. Wisseman's leadership, in 1962, and progressed through the ranks to full professor in 1983. Traub, while at WRAIR, was a key member of the scrub typhus group in Kuala Lumpur, Malaya in 1948. His work was largely instrumental in the successful chemoprophylaxis studies of scrub typhus. Traub and the entomology team identified and pinpointed the field test area where exposure to typhus-infected mites was conducted. Later they showed and reported the existence of small foci of typhus-infected mites (mite island) in indigenous rodents and chiggers which varied significantly after several years, based on ecologic considerations. Also identified were new chiggers, major vectors of scrub typhus. A significant study revealed the successful use of Dieldrin as an effective means of ground control of mites.[7-15]

Dr. Traub retired from the academic faculty in 1983 and assumed the important position of Honorary Curator (Fleas) at the Smithsonian Institute.

With his associate Abdu Azad, they showed for the first time that fleas can transmit the agent of murine typhus (*Rickettsia typhi*) by the bite as well as contamination of the bite wound with infected feces. Also, they made the initial report that *R. typhi* may be transovarially transmitted in fleas, thus extending the common feature that maintains murine typhus rickettsiae in nature.[16] Moreover, their ecological studies of murine typhus in highlands of Ethiopia and Burma revealed the involvement

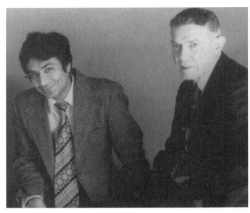

Abdu F. Azad, Ph.D. and Robert Traub, Ph.D.

of indoor rats and their fleas in the maintenance of the *R. typhi* cycle. Extension of murine typhus studies in endemic areas of the United States, namely, southern Texas and Los Angeles County, California, resulted in the discovery of a new murine typhus-like rickettsial species (*R. felis*).[17] Azad and Traub also showed that the common fleas found on cats and dogs can transmit murine typhus rickettsia.[18,19]

Andrew (Andy) Smith, who joined the Department of Microbiology in 1950, gave great strength to the laboratory teaching program for students and fellows. From 1972 until 1983 when he retired, Andy directed the Division of Microbiology of the Department of Pathology, in the clinical laboratories of the hospital. He was an authoritative source for mycologic problems and sparked the entire microbiologic diagnostic service. Joint academic professional appointments were held in medicine, dermatology, and pathology. His many solid publications focused on serodiagnosis and therapy of fungal infections and early diagnostic techniques. He served as President of the American Society of Microbiology, Maryland (1961), and the University of Maryland Biological Society (1962–1963).

Q FEVER

Our interest in Q fever dated from the early 1950s involving chemotherapy of rickettsial diseases. Dr. Hornick later worked at the Rocky Mountain Spotted Fever Laboratory in Hamilton where he gained extensive experience with naturally occurring cases of the illness. He also learned the use and limitations of the skin test and vaccines.

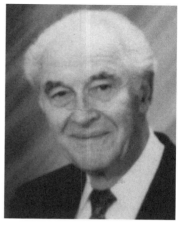

Andrew Smith, Ph.D.

Dr. Paul Fiset joined the faculty in 1964, in microbiology, under Dr. Wisseman. He was elevated to the rank of professor in 1974. His pioneering work led to characterization of Q fever rickettsiae (*Coxiella burnetii*) and revealed two antigenic phases, I and II. He began this work with his associate Dr. M.G.P. Stoker while working in Cambridge, England.[20] Fiset pursued this work throughout his career which was of great significance in helping develop new knowledge pertaining to better means of detection and control of Q fever by immunization.

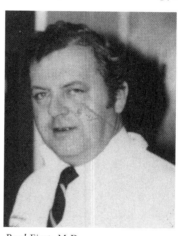

Paul Fiset, M.D.

Dr. William Tigertt, former Commandant at USAMRIID (Ft. Detrick) and WRAIR (Bethesda), joined our faculty as Professor of Pathology and Head of the Clinical Laboratories in 1970. While at Ft. Detrick, he and his associate, Dr. Abram Benenson, determined the human infectious dose of *C. burnetii*, and showed that available vaccines protected against illness after aerosol exposure to viable pathogenic Q fever rickettsiae.[21] Division members collaborated in these studies which were an important part

of the BW control and volunteer programs. Our group, led by
Bert DuPont, showed that the living Q fever vaccine did not lead
to troublesome hepatic granuloma formation.[22,23]

ROCKY MOUNTAIN SPOTTED FEVER

Persistence of Viable Rickettsiae in Convalescent Patient with RMSF

Hans Zinsser of Harvard surmised that recurrent typhus fever,
many years after the initial infection (Brills disease), was ex-
plained on the basis that rickettsiae persisted in a viable but qui-
escent state and occasionally re-emerged to cause a second active
but milder infection. We approached this hypothesis by carefully
studying a patient who was extremely ill with RMSF and who
fully recovered. About 14 months after his recovery, we removed
an inguinal lymph gland to test for the presence of viable rickettsiae knowing that if any were present, they would be few in
number. Guinea pigs were given large doses of prednisone to suppress their immune system. One half of the lymph node was injected intraperitoneally into two guinea pigs. They developed
fever for about a week and living pathogenic rickettsiae were
demonstrated in these animals; the agent was transferred to other
animals. This simply confirmed Zinsser's remarkable wisdom
regarding microbial persistence.

First Identification of Rickettsia in Skin Specimen of RMSF Patient by Immunofluoresence

In order to approach the problem of laboratory confirmation
during the early stages of RMSF, we attacked the issue directly.
After all, headache, fever, myalgia, and rash (the hallmark of
RMSF) can be confused with other acute infections. Diagnosis by
demonstration of proteus agglutinins or antibody, of necessity,
comes later, often when the patient has either recovered or died.
Rickettsial diseases are vasculitides, and, as Wolbach showed
years before, the causative rickettsiae are in endothelial cells.
However, their identification by staining and microscopy was difficult. The newer technique of immunofluorescence, first described by Dr. Albert Coons, which visualized antigen or antibody in infected animal tissues, afforded the ideal opportunity. In
1976, we obtained a small piece of skin taken at the site of a pink

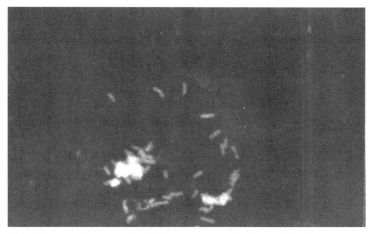

Skin biopsy: rickettsia of Rocky Mountain spotted fever (RMSF) by immune peroxidase method (1976)

macular lesion of a child on the third day of RMSF. Using fluorescein and specific antibody under dark field microscopy, specific rickettsiae were easily visualized. The whole procedure took about 3½ hours.[25] Now this is standard procedure in many centers and is a great help in early diagnostic confirmation.

Transmission of RMSF by Blood Transfusion

In 1978, it was shown that the rickettsiae of RMSF were transmitted by blood taken from a patient as a blood donor during the incubation period.[26] The donor, not knowing of the infection at the time, later developed RMSF. The recipient of the blood who developed classic RMSF was hospitalized at the Maryland General Hospital. His blood yielded pathogenic *R. rickettsii* which was confirmed by animal inoculation. The recipient of the contaminated blood recovered fully with treatment.

Vaccine Efficacy Testing of RMSF in Volunteers

From the early 20th century following the work of Ricketts, Spencer, and Parker, there was controversy regarding the actual efficacy of vaccine against RMSF. The first product was derived from tick tissues and was accompanied by severe, local reactions. Later vaccines developed by Cox, using the chicken embryo technique to grow rickettsiae, appeared to be more protective and unaccompanied by severe reactions. However, its protective efficacy appeared to be limited. As new vaccines became available, including a concentrated product comprised of many rickettsiae grown in tissue cultures, trials were conducted in volunteers to determine the true effect. Controlled studies showed that the vaccines protected against severe illness and those who became ill had milder illnesses than the uninoculated. Also in some vaccinees who becaume ill, the incubation period tended to be longer.[27,28] These studies performed in collaboration with associates at Ft. Detrick clarified this problem which had long been under question.

In 1979, Mary Lou Clements joined the Department of Medicine as Assistant Professor of Medicine and the Chief of the Clinical Studies Section of the Center for Vaccine Development. Her careful studies with others, in volunteers, helped clarify the long-standing controversy regarding efficacy of older and current vaccines for RMSF. Her investigative work on oral rehydration for dehydrated patients and vaccine evaluation of important enteric pathogens such as V. cholera and E. coli was outstanding.[29] In 1985, she returned to the Johns Hopkins University School of Hygiene and Public Health where she became Associate

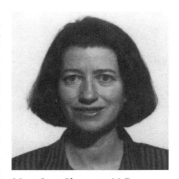

Mary Lou Clements, M.D.

Professor of International Health and Director of the Center for Immunization Research.

J. Stephen Dumler, a 1985 graduate of the University of Maryland School of Medicine, trained in pathology and laboratory medicine in the Department of Pathology, Johns Hopkins University School of Medicine, 1985–1990, and as a postdoctoral fellow and instructor with Dr. David Walker at the University of Texas, Medical Branch, Galveston, 1990–1992. From 1992 to 1995, Dr. Dumler was Assistant Professor of Pathology at the University of Maryland School of Medicine and Associate Director of the University Hospital Microbiology Laboratory. He was appointed to the Hopkins faculty in 1996, where he is Associate Professor of Pathology and Director, Division of Medical Microbiology. His research contributions are impressive, and at this early age, he is one of America's leading authorities on rickettsial diseases and other vector-borne illnesses such as Ehrlichosis and Lyme borreliosis. While at Maryland, he worked closely with Dr. Wisseman and associates in the Department of Microbiology and with others in the Department of Medicine.

His seminal work included newer methods of serodiagnosis and other immunologic procedures for RMSF, classic evaluation of available vaccines for prevention of RMSF in volunteers, development of newer techniques for early diagnosis of causative rickettsiae in skin and other tissues using immunoperoxidase methods. Further work elucidated and characterized cell-mediated immune reactions and the nature of the inflammatory process in epidemic typhus as well as the spotted fevers.[30-38]

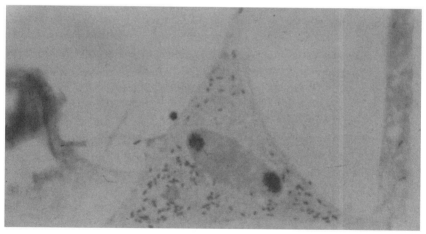

Rickettsia of RMSF by tissue culture (Wisseman et al.)

REFERENCES

1. Pincoffs MC, Guy EB, Lister LM, Woodward TE, Smadel JE. The treatment of Rocky Mountain spotted fever with Chloromycetin. Ann Intern Med 1948;29:656–663.

2. Woodward TE, Blanc EJ. Clinical observations in typhus fever with special reference to the cardiovascular system. JAMA 1944;126: 287–293.

3. Workman JB, Hightower JA, Borges FJ, Furman JHE, Parker RT. Cortisone as an adjunct to chloramphenicol in the treatment of Rocky Mountain spotted fever. N Engl J Med 1962;246:962.

4. Wisseman CL Jr, Jackson EM, Hahn FE, Ley HL, Smadel JE. The effects of antimicrobial substance and enzyme inhibition of the oxidation of glutamate by purified rickettsiae. J Immunol 1951;67:123.

5. Patterson PY, Wisseman CL Jr, Smadel JE. Studies of rickettsial toxins. I. Role of hemolysis in fatal toxemia of rabbits and rats. J. Immunol 1954;72:12.

6. Wattenberg LE, Wisseman CL Jr, Smadel JE. Studies of rickettsial toxins. II. Altered vascular physiology in rickettsial toxemia in mice. J Immunol 1956;74:147.

7. Philip CB, Traub R, Smadel JE. Chloramphenicol (Chloromycetin) in the chemoprophylaxis of scrub typhus (tsutsugamushi disease). I. Epidemiological observations in hyperendemic areas of scrub typhus in Malaya. Am J Hyg 1949;50(1):63–74.

8. Traub R, Wisseman CL Jr. The ecology of chigger-borne rickettsioses (scrub typhus). J Med Entomol 11 1974;(3):237–303.

9. Traub R, Frick LP, Diercks FH. Observations on the occurrence of rickettsia tsutsugamushi in rats and mites in the Malayan jungle. Am J Hyg 1950;51(3):269–273.

10. Traub R, Wisseman CL Jr. Ecological considerations in scrub typhus. I. Emerging concepts. Bull WHO 1968;39(2):209–218.

11. Traub R. Some considerations of mites and ticks as vectors of human disease. In Proceedings of the Symposium on Biological Transmission of Disease Agents. Academic Press: New York, 1962, pp. 123–134.

12. Traub R, Wisseman CL Jr. Ecological considerations in scrub typhus. II. Vector-species. Bull WHO 1968;39(2):219–230.

13. Traub R, Wisseman CL Jr. Current concepts of the ecology of chigger-borne rickettsiosis (scrub typhus). Jpn J Med Sci Biol 1974; 1:1–5.

14. Traub R, Newson HD, Walton BC, Audy JR. Efficacy of Dieldrin and Aldrin in area control of the chigger vectors of scrub typhus. J Econ Entomol 1954;47(3):429–435.

15. Traub R, Dowling MAC. The duration of efficacy of the insecticide Dieldrin against the chigger vectors of scrub typhus in Malaya. J Econ Entomol 1961;54(4):654–659.

16. Azad AF, Sacci FB, Nelson WM, Dasch CA, Schmidman ET, Carl M. Genetic characterization and transovarial transmission of a novel typhus-like rickettsia found in cat fleas. Proc Natl Acad Sci USA 1992; 89:43–46.

17. Higgins JA, Radulovic S, Schriefer ME, Azad AF. *Rickettsia felis*: a new species of pathogenic rickettsia isolated from cat fleas. J Clin Microbiol 1996;34:671–74.

18. Azad AR, Traub R. Experimental transmission of murine typhus by *Xenopsylla cheopis* flea bites. Med Vet Entomol 1989;3:429–433.

19. Farhang-Azad A, Traub R, Baqar S. Transovarial transmission of murine typhus rickettsiae in *Xenopsylla cheopis* fleas. Science 227(4686): 543–545, 1985.

20. Stoker MGP, Fiset P. Phase variation of the Nine Mile fever and other strains of *Rickettsia burnetii*. Can. J. Microbiol. 1956;2:310–321.

21. Tigertt WB, Benenson AS. Studies on Q fever in man. Trans Assoc Am Physicians 1956;69:98–104.

22. Dupont HL, Hornick RB, Levin HS, Rapport MI, Woodward TE. Q fever hepatitis. Ann Intern Med 1971;74:148.

23. Woodward TE, Ricketts AL. Diseases with emphasis upon Rocky Mountain spotted fever and Q fever. Proc Int Symp South Africa, Capetown, 1977:450–470.

24. Parker RT, Menon PG, Merideth AM, Snyder MJ, Woodward TE. Persistence of rickettsia Rickettsii in a patient recovered from Rocky Mountain spotted fever. J Immunol 1954;73:383–386.

25. Woodward TE, Pederson CE Jr, Oster CN, Bagley LR, Romberger J, Snyder MJ. Prompt confirmation of Rocky Mountain spotted fever: Identification of rickettsiae in skin tissues. J Infect Dis 1976; 134:296.

26. Wells GM, Woodward TE, Fiset P, Hornick RB. Rocky Mountain spotted fever caused by blood transfusions. JAMA 1978;239: 2763–2765.

27. Archer MS, Oster CN, Harber PI, Kenyon RH, Pedersen CE Jr. Initial clinical evaluation of a new Rocky Mountain spotted fever vaccine of tissue culture origin. J Infect Dis 1978;138:217–221.

28. Dupont HL, Hornick RB, Dawkins AT, Heiner GG, Fabrikant IB, Wisseman CL Jr, Woodward TE. Rocky Mountain spotted fever: a comparative study of the active immunity induced by inactivated and viable pathogenic *Rickettsia rickettsii*. J Infect Dis 1973;128,340–344.

29. Clements ML, Wisseman CL Jr, Woodward TE, Fiset P, Dumler JS, McNamee W, Black RE, Rooney J, Hughes TP, Levine MM. Reactogenicity, immunogenicity and efficacy of a chick embryo cell-derived vaccine for Rocky Mountain spotted fever. J Infect Dis 1983;148: 922–930.

30. Clements ML, Dumler JS, Fiset P, Wisseman CL Jr, Snyder MJ, Levine MM. Serodiagnosis of Rocky Mountain spotted fever: Comparison of IgM and IgG enzyme-linked immunosorbent assay and indirect fluorescent antibody test. J Infect Dis 1983;148:876–880.

31. Clements ML, Wisseman CL Jr, Woodward TE, Fiset P, Dumler JS, McNamee W, Black RE, Rooney J, Hughes TP, Levine MM. Reactogenicity, immunogenicity, and efficacy of a chick embryo cell-derived vaccine for Rocky Mountain spotted fever. J Infect Dis 1983;148: 922–930.

32. Dumler JS, Gage WR, Pettis GL, Azad AF, Kuhajda FP. Rapid immunoperoxidase demonstration of *Rickettsia rickettsii* in fixed cutaneous specimens in patients with Rocky Mountain spotted fever. Am J Clin Pathol 1990;93:410–414.

33. Dumler JS, Wisseman CL Jr, Fiset P, Clements ML. Cell-mediated immune responses of adults to vaccination, challenge with *Rickettsia rickettsii*, or both. Am J Trop Med Hyg 1992;46:105–115.

34. Dumler JS, Wisseman CL Jr. Preliminary characterization of inflammatory infiltrates in response to *Rickettsia prowazekii* reinfection in man: Immunohistology. Acta Virol 1992;36:45–51.

35. Woodward TE, Dumler JS, Walker DH. The remarkable contributions of S. Burt Wolbach on rickettsial vasculitis updated. Trans Am Clin Climatol Assoc 1991;103:78–94.

36. Clements ML, Dumler JS, Fiset P, Levine MM, Woodward TE. Serodiagnosis of Rocky Mountain spotted fever: Current status. American College of Physicians, Regional Meeting, Baltimore, MD, August 1982.

37. Dumler JS, Wisseman CL Jr, Fiset P, Clements ML. Cell mediated immunity in volunteers who were vaccinated, challenged with virulent *Rickettsia rickettsii*, or both. Eighth Sesqui-Annual Meeting of the American Society for Rickettsiology and Rickettsial Diseases, Diamond Point, NY, September 1989.

38. Dumler JS, Wisseman CL Jr. Preliminary characterization of inflammatory infiltrates in response to intradermal *Rickettsia prowazekii* reinfection in man: Immunohistology. IVth International Symposium on Rickettsiae and Rickettsial Diseases, Piestany, Czechoslovakia, October 1990.

7

MENINGITIS

Theodore E. Woodward, M.D.

Even now at the end of the 20th century, and after about 65 years use of specific antibacterial chemotherapy, pyrogenic meningitis continues to take a significant toll. There are reasons for this. In 1944 Dr. Worth Daniels, Sr., a distinguished Washington physician, commented, "Meningococci may attack so subtly as to elude diagnosis and so rapidly as to out-distance treatment." Acute fulminant meningococcemia fits this description, and meningococcal meningitis can progress very rapidly. Pneumococci can rapidly cause devastating meningitis and many other serious problems. The failures today result from delay in diagnosis and institution of proper therapy by the right doses and routes, and the inability to fully reverse the deleterious early inflammatory alterations caused by bacteria or their toxins. Now there is the specter of resistance to antibiotic activity.

I recall as a medical student in 1939 that Dr. James (Jake) Arnold, a leading Baltimore neurologist, and our teacher, successfully treated a child with streptococcal meningitis with sulfonamide at the Church Home and Hospital. This result, the first, seemed like a miracle. Later, Dr. Arnold became one of Baltimore's leading neurosurgeons.

University of Maryland's entry into this important field really began in 1948, after the broad-range effects of Aureomycin (tetracycline) and chloramphenicol were realized. At the time, penicillin, which came into general use after WW II, was effective in meningitis caused by meningococci, pneumococci, and beta streptococci. It had no helpful action in *Hemophilus influenzae* meningitis so prevalent in children. Moreover, the blood–brain barrier for penicillin was a definite limitation. Lepper and Dowling, then working in Chicago, stressed the need for meningeal doses of penicillin which required approximately 20 million units given intravenously daily for effective treatment. They also later reported that broad-spectrum antibiotics, specifically Aureomycin, given simultaneously with penicillin were antagonistic and deleterious, rather than helpful. This combination study was not carefully controlled, but had great influence on medical practice.

During the early 20th century, immune sera were used for the major types of meningitis, and later serum treatment was used in combination with sulfonamide and some of the newer antibiotics. Sulfonamides proved very effective for meningococcal meningitis, but unfortunately, drug resistance later developed.

We began our studies in 1948 with the opportunity to treat patients at the University and Mercy Hospitals, in other Baltimore hospitals, and at our research units in Puerto Rico and Pakistan. We enjoyed full support and collaboration with Dr. Ed Bradley and our pediatric colleagues at the University Hospital. Various physicians throughout the country, and pediatricians in particular, were then utilizing multiple antibiotic regimens for children with meningitis, on the premise that if one is good, two are better, and so on. The common combinations were penicillin with a sulfonamide and either tetracycline or chloramphenicol, or even a combination of the latter two. Jawetz in California had reported antagonistic action in vitro when a group I bactericidal antibiotic (penicillin, streptomycin) was combined with a group II bacteriostatic antibiotic (tetracycline, chloramphenicol). The suppressive effect of the bacteriostatic antibiotic was thought to deny the bactericidal antibiotic its proper setting for action during the logarithmic stage of bacterial growth. Sulfonamides were classified as suppressive in action (group II). These facts appeared to be true in the test tube, but were not fully corroborated in humans when varying doses or differing times of administering antibiotics were utilized.

At this time, it was realized that about 80% of all of the acute meningitides (excluding tuberculosis) were caused by meningococci, pneumococci, and *H. influenzae*. The dilemma regarding treatment stimulated our interest and prompted the clinical trials to find other answers to simplify therapy. We surmised that if an orally administered antibiotic with a wide range of antibacterial action could produce adequate levels in the blood and cerebrospinal fluid (CSF), much advantage could be gained. Moreover, in a setting with limited facilities such as in a remote village or rural area, oral antibiotic treatment of meningitis might be readily available and life-saving. Unfortunately, in many remote areas, a spinal puncture is impractical. Obviously, the pharmacologic features for the new antibiotics needed to be fully ascertained to determine whether *only one* broad-spectrum antibiotic could suffice for treatment of meningitis. These were the practical objectives, and the results were perceived as potentially useful in the academic center.

In Baltimore, after WW II, patients, including children, with acute infectious diseases such as diphtheria, scarlet fever, meningitis, mumps, typhoid, and rheumatic fever, were admitted to the Sydenham Hospital in North Baltimore. It was located on Lake Montebello near the Memorial stadium. It later became the Montebello State Hospital for chronic illness and rehabilitation. Dr. Julius M. Waghlestein, an internist, and Dr. Francis Schwentker, a distinguished Hopkins pediatrician, were Scientific Directors at Sydenham. Many of us went there to work with patients. With the explosion of new antibiotics in 1948, and thereafter, most hospitals improved their isolation procedures so that patients could be handled in adequately appointed units with little threat of spread from person to person. Also, procedures for cardiovascular, respiratory, renal, and circulatory support needed in seriously ill patients with infectious diseases were readily accessible.

At the time, in Baltimore, we believed that we were the first to successfully treat children and adults with meningitis using one broad-spectrum antibiotic. The use of one drug would clearly define clinical action of a specific antibiotic and avoid the issue of antagonism or the need for additive help from other medications.

It was found that tetracycline and chloramphenicol absorbed well from the upper GI tract within about 30 minutes. Good blood levels occurred, and each antibiotic diffused into the subarachnoid space with very effective levels in the CSF. Also, antibiotic concentrations were high in the urine and bile. It was anticipated that critically ill and comatose patients with meningitis would require intravenous treatment in order for the antibiotic to reach the target area (brain and meninges) as soon as possible. Dosage schedules were ultimately based on kilograms per body weight; tetracycline (25 mg/kg) and chloramphenicol (50 mg/kg) were used as the initial large loading dose, and the daily doses were administered orally and given in divided doses at 6- or 8-hour intervals. In some situations, either of these broad-spectrum antibiotics could be dissolved and given by gastric tube when IV fluids were unavailable, or when patients could not swallow.

Based on promising in vitro evidence, we began treatment of children with *H. influenzae* meningitis in 1949.[1] Response to treatment was prompt, and in seven patients observed in 1949–1950, the results were excellent. Clinical manifestations were markedly better in 36 hours, and fever abated in an average of 3 days. When treatment was initiated soon after onset of illness, recovery was complete without residual effects. Delay in starting specific treatment for a day or so was followed occasionally by continuing eye signs, lingering irritability, or behavioral changes. These usually ultimately abated.

Soon to follow were commendable results with chloramphenicol based on 17 treated cases.[2] Death occurred in two children whose treatment was initiated late in illness at critical stages: coma in one and serious neurologic manifestations and a superimposed infection in another. During these early trials, Dr. Margaret Smith of New Orleans visited Baltimore, and we had the opportunity to discuss these early results with her. She made an excellent study and published the initial report.

Soon after oral administration of either tetracycline or chloramphenicol, blood and CSF levels with antibiotic were achieved within an hour and often earlier. Later, a liquid form of chloramphenicol (Palmitate) was shown to absorb well from the GI tract with ultimately adequate blood and CSF concentrations.[3] Caution was needed to shake the liquid emulsion well, since the antibiotic seemed to settle in the container.

Each of the broad-spectrum antibiotics (tetracycline and chloramphenicol) was shown to be solely effective in the treatment of meningococcal and pneumococcal meningitis.[4-6]

There were some fatalities and complications as is always the case in critically ill patients. Specifically, of 62 patients with meningococcal meningitis treated with chloramphenicol, there was one death (2.0%); 61 patients recovered fully. In the lethal case, there were bilateral adrenal hemorrhages.

Using chloramphenicol alone, 36 patients with pneumococcal meningitis recovered, and 4 patients died (11%). Several patients died within an hour or so of hospitalization. These results compared favorably with other reported treatment regimens, particularly with penicillin.

A total of 35 patients with *H. influenzae* meningitis were treated solely with chloramphenicol from 1950 to 1965; 32 recovered fully, and 3 died (7%) as a consequence of treatment being first initiated at a critical stage with serious neurologic signs.

Sporadic cases of specific types of meningitis caused by other organisms and treated solely with chloramphenicol were *Salmonella choleraesuis, Listeria monocytogenes*, hemolytic staphylococci, *Streptococcus viridans*, beta hemolytic streptococcus, and nonhemolytic streptococcus; all recovered.

The point was simply made by us that conventional and standard regimens should be utilized, and that tetracycline and chloramphenicol were effective backup agents for meningitis. In influenzal meningitis, they should be regarded as indicated methods of treatment. Also, these findings were regarded as potentially useful for treatment of patients with presumed bacterial meningitis in whom the agent was not specifically identified.[7-8]

REFERENCES

1. Drake ME, Bradley JE, Imburg J, McCrumb FR Jr, Woodward TE. Aureomycin in the treatment of influenzal meningitis. JAMA 1950;142:463–465.

2. McCrumb FR Jr, Hall HE, Imburg J, Meredith A, Helmhold R, Defillo JB, Woodward TE. Treatment of hemophilus influenzae meningitis with chloramphenicol and other antibiotics. JAMA 1951;145:469–474.

3. Deane GE, Furman JE, Bentz AO, Woodward TE. Treatment of meningitis with Chloromycetin Palmitate: Results of therapy in twenty-three cases. Pediatrics 1953;11:368–380.

4. McCrumb FR Jr, Hall HE, Merideth A, Deane GE, Minor JV Jr, Woodward TE. Chloramphenicol in the treatment of meningococcal meningitis. Am J Med 1951;10:696–703.

5. Menon PG, Raskin JF, Woodward TE. Further experience with chloramphenicol in treatment of meningococcal meningitis. Antibiotics and Chemotherapy, 1954;4:1113–1116.

6. Parker RT, Snyder MJ, Liu RSJ, Looper JW Jr, Woodward TE. Therapeutic range of chloramphenicol in purulent meningitis. Antibiotics Annual, 1954–1955. New York Medical Encyclopedia, Inc., 1955, pp. 26–34.

7. Hornick RB, Gallager LR, Ronald AR, Abdullah J, Khan MA, Khan I, Hassan S, Messer J, Shafi MJ, Ud-Din Z, Woodward, TE. Chloramphenicol treatment of pyrogenic meningitis. Bull School Med Univ Maryland 1966;51:43.

8. Rapoport MI, Woodward TE. Neurologic emergencies. Pyrogenic meningitis. Emergency room care. The Thirty-third Hahnemann Symposium by Grune & Stratton, Inc., 1972.

8

EARLY STUDIES ON TULAREMIA AND PLAGUE

Theodore E. Woodward, M.D.

During the 1930s and early 1940s, tularemia was a common disorder with frequent hospitalization of patients, particularly from rural areas. It also involved city residents. I recall, as a medical student, walking to school via the Lexington Market and noting wild rabbits, dressed, hanging, and ready for sale with yellowish white spots showing on their livers and abdominal contents (caseous granulomas). Butchers frequently contracted the disease, as well as wives of hunters who had cleaned rabbits killed by their husbands. Of local interest, Dr. Huntington Williams, the Baltimore City Commissioner of Health, noted the high incidence of tularemia in the city. In about 1938, he practically single-handedly forced the City Council to pass an ordinance to prohibit the sale of wild cotton-tailed rabbits in Baltimore. The infection rate in Baltimore dropped sharply.

Several types of clinical infection occurred: 1) ulceroglandular, which was usually clinically mild; 2) a bacteremic form that resembled typhoid fever and carried a significant fatality rate; 3) tularemic pneumonia, which was about 30% fatal; and 4) oculoglandular, a very severe type of infection. Diagnosis was made from the epidemiologic history, particularly involving contact with rabbits; clinical manifestations; isolation of *Pasteurella tularensis* by culture, which was difficult; and isolation by animal inoculation (guinea pigs), a hazardous laboratory procedure. The agglutination test was a reliable confirmatory procedure and became definitely positive by about the 14th day of illness. Smears of ulcerative lesions occasionally revealed Gram-negative intracellular bacteria.

The first effective treatment was streptomycin, which became available in 1949. Para-aminobenzoic acid was only moderately beneficial, and sulfonamide and penicillin were not useful; however, the action of streptomycin was dramatic. Unfortunately, it had to be given by injection and was accompanied by serious side effects, and it was not effective orally. In 1948, in this setting, we began studies of tularemia, particularly when it was found that Chloromycetin and Aureomycin were active against rickettsia.[1,2] They are obligate intracellular organisms resembling *P. tularensis* in some ways.

Animal studies in guinea pigs and mice performed largely by Bob Parker, Merrill Snyder, Leonard Lister, Robert Bauer, Howard Hall, and Ann Meredith showed that the tetracycline antibiotics (Aureomycin) and Chloromycetin effectively controlled the infection. The action of these broad-spectrum antibiotics was through bacteriostatic and nonbactericidal mechanisms of action. Relapses occurred when antibiotic therapy was initiated very early in the illness (similar to the experience in scrub typhus fever when treatment was initiated before the 5th febrile day). Fortunately, antibiotic resistance to *P. tularensis* did not develop, and treatment led to a prompt response. These studies represented improvement simply because these medications were effective when given *orally* as well as intravenously when needed in seriously ill patients. *P. tularensis* was then regarded as a potential biologic warfare agent. Russian scientists, then active in the field, had developed an effective viable vaccine for protection against tularemia. These realizations had relevance regarding the status of plague, a recognized biologic threat.

STUDIES OF TULAREMIA IN VOLUNTEERS

After the promising results of animal studies, the important questions were whether infection in humans could be induced by aerosol exposure and determination of the infectious dose. It was also necessary to evaluate the actual efficacy of the available antibiotics. Also the protective effects of the tularemic vaccines merited evaluation. Monkeys exposed, by inhalation, to relatively few living *P. tularensis* organisms, in specially prepared dispensers at USA MRIID (Fort Detrick), developed pneumonia by this method. Antibiotic therapy was quite effective. We then prepared a proposal for human testing to be performed under our auspices to address the aforementioned problems.

All contemplated testing in volunteers was subject to peer review with careful scrutiny and approval by the Commissions of Epidemiologic Survey and Immunization of the AFEB and the Board itself. The Department of Defense ultimately approved and funded the study.

It was not possible to transport Maryland prison inmate volunteers to a federal agency such as Ft. Detrick. A special trailer (mobile) laboratory chamber was constructed and taken to the Maryland Correctional Institution at Jessup, Maryland, where we had established a strong affiliation. Inmates volunteered willingly, without coercion or any inducements such as financial rewards or lessening of their prison terms. They were fully informed of all possible medical developments (see Chapter 14).

After thorough screening and evaluation of the health status of each individual, the study was initiated. After their infection was induced by the special respiratory dispenser, volunteers were taken immediately to the newly developed medical care unit at Jessup manned by physicians, nurses, and key personnel. All activities were carefully monitored by senior infectious disease personnel and included medical residents and students along with medical scientists of USA MRIID. Fortunately, there were no serious adverse manifestations in volunteers, morale was high, and much new and valuable information was acquired. Col. William Tigertt, M.C., and Col. Daniel Crozier, M.C., Commanders of USA MRIID, were staunch helpful planners, collaborators, and supporters. Each carried faculty appointments in the Department of Medicine. Dr. Henry T. Eiglesbach, MB Division, Ft. Detrick, prepared the challenge and vaccine strains and performed many informative experimental studies in animals.

The results showed that tularemic infection was induced in humans by aerosolization of a few pathogenic *P. tularensis* organisms. They also indicated that 1) a pneumonic infection could be visual-

ized by chest x-ray; 2) early therapy with streptomycin, tetracycline, or chloramphenicol was effective clinically[3]; 3) Russian-type
viable vaccine which was purified at USA MRIID, given intrader-
mally, afforded effective protection against aerosol exposure tularemia; and 4) intradermal vaccination prevented systemic infection and only a small local reaction developed.

The findings had considerable relevance regarding the status
of plague, a recognized biologic threat.

PLAGUE

In 1950–1951, plague was high on the list of biologic weapons,
simply because this human illness can be devastating and incite
panic. Furthermore, interest along these lines was increased because a strange vaccine was encountered in North Korea when
General Douglas MacArthur's forces reached the Yalu River on
the border of Korea and China. Several communist hospital units
were captured intact; among the medical equipment were vials of
a vaccine labeled "E.V. plague." The bacterial contents was pack-
aged and dried in sealed vials. This, itself, indicated that plague
was a potential threat. There were confirmed reports that Japanese scientists had actively engaged in plague research during
WW II and actively tried it as a biologic weapon in China. Samples of vaccines were conveyed to Dr. Karl Meyer, Director of the
Hooper Foundation in San Francisco. Meyer, then considered
America's Pasteur, was one of the world's authorities on plague.
The captured dried vaccine, dissolved in liquid culture media,
was found to be viable with living plague bacilli. This feat had
not been accomplished in America previously.

E.V. plague was known as an avirulent plague strain first isolated from a patient with bubonic plague in Madagascar by Dr.
G. Girard (a French plague expert). The initials of the patient
from whom the vaccine was made were E.V. Originally virulent,
after numerous passages in culture media, it became nonvirulent
and viable. Girard developed a living vaccine from this strain at
the Pasteur Institute, Paris. Although it produced a local dermal
reaction, similar to smallpox vaccine virus, it was used effectively
in endemic plague countries to protect against the "Black Death."

Joe Smadel, Ken Goodner, and Woodward discussed how we
might protect against such lethal illness if a dried virulent aerosol
was dispersed over a wide area. One virulent bacterium could in-

fect a human. An explosive device could possibly set a pneumonic plague outbreak immediately in motion.

In 1951, the only known reliable treatment for any type of plague was streptomycin. Sulfonamides had only weak action. Streptomycin had to be injected twice daily, posing a huge logistic problem for management of any large population group. Obviously, an orally administered antibiotic would be of great advantage.

Tularemia and plague have common features clinically including: fever, great prostration, enlarged lymph glands (buboes), and pneumonia. This last feature is usually fatal without treatment. Plague could be regarded as simply tularemia multiplied in severity about three times. We, therefore, wondered whether the newer broad-spectrum antibiotics, Chloromycetin and Aureomycin (tetracycline), given orally would cure plague. We had determined experimentally in Baltimore that in guinea pigs, mice, and humans, these antibiotics cured tularemia about as effectively as streptomycin. Experimental work on plague was prohibited in the eastern United States simply because plague was not endemic there. Some work was permitted at Ft. Detrick where in vitro testing with the newer antibiotics showed some inhibitory action against *P. pestis* (plague).

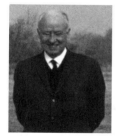

We concluded, with AFEB concurrence, that a reliable and practical treatment of human plague was required. Joe Smadel, then Scientific Director at WRAIR, consulted with Dr. James H.S. Gear, a senior scientist at the South African Institute for Medical Research in Johannesburg. Gear had worked at the Rockefeller Institute during the war and knew Smadel and Goodner. Plague was prevalent in South Africa, and an invitation to visit followed. Gear indicated that small but sizeable outbreaks of plague occurred sporadically in African natives (Bantu) throughout the country. En route to Johannesburg, we stopped in Paris to meet and talk with Dr. Girard at the Pasteur Institute. We learned much about plague from him.

Dr. James H.S. Gear

On arrival in Johannesburg, we learned that a sizeable outbreak of plague in a Bantu village, which we had planned to evaluate, had subsided. This precluded the chance for a treatment trial. Many natives in the villages died of pneumonic plague—a tragic experience.

Although this chance for a therapeutic trial eluded us, Dr. Girard had suggested a visit to Madagascar and had graciously arranged a visit with Dr. J. Robic, Director of the Pasteur Institute in Tannarive. This was only a slight detour from Johannesburg. Dr. Robic received us hospitably and arranged meetings with appropriate public health officials. Plague is endemic in this mountainous island. Rats abound in this primitive rural country, and the rat–fleas–human plague cycle is a natural epidemiologic fact. Once bubonic plague occurs, septicemic and pneumonic plague soon follow. Patients with human plague were located within a short distance from the Pasteur Institute. We were taken to observe acute plague cases, allowed to examine them carefully, and treat a few sputum-positive confirmed patients, including pneumonic and bacteremic types. We used chloramphenicol first and found that if antibiotic treatment was given sufficiently early in illness, the response was excellent, similar to that following streptomycin treatment.[4] Although the limited studies were encouraging, there were insufficient numbers of patients to convincingly prove the point statistically. Conjecture or a promising lead is inadequate.

Based on the preliminary favorable clues, we returned to America determined to finish the objective. A grant from the De-

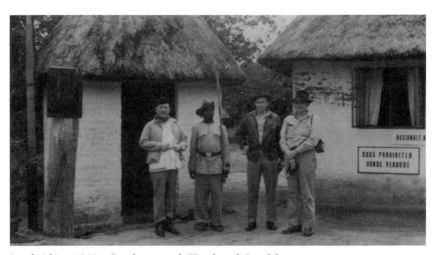

South Africa, 1951—Goodner, guard, Woodward, Smadel

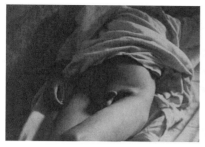

Bubonic plague. Note enlarged inguinal bubo.

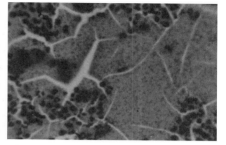

Plague (smear of bubo)

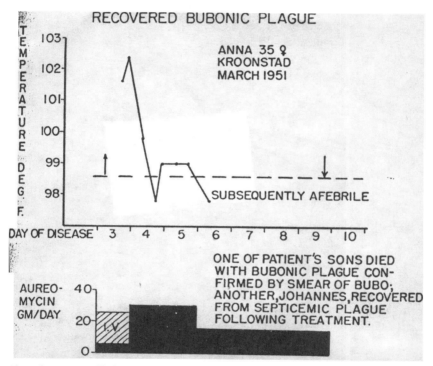

Clinical response of bubonic plague patient to Aureomycin therapy

partment of Defense to the Department of Medicine (Infectious Diseases) enabled completion of the study. We selected Dr. Fred McCrumb to complete the clinical investigation of plague. He first went to the Hooper Foundation with K.F. Meyer in San Francisco, performed extensive studies on antibiotic efficacy in plague-infected monkeys, and learned the immunologic characteristics of the bacillus. Mc-Crumb took a language instruction course in French in preparation for his visit to Madagascar in order to complete the study with the Pasteur group. Carefully designed studies in patients with pneumonic plague confirmed bacteriologically that chloramphenicol and tetracycline (Aureomycin) cured patients just as effectively as streptomycin.[5] However, to be curative, any of the three antibiotics (Chloromycetin, tetracycline, or streptomycin) needed to be given not later

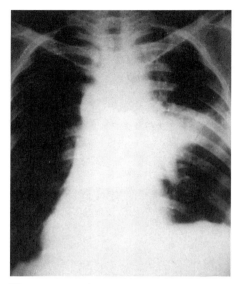

Plague pneumonia

than about 20 hours from the onset of illness. The plague toxin is potent. Hence, the oral route of therapy proved to be a potentially effective approach for control, involving large numbers of patients.[6]

Much later we derived some satisfaction from hearing of the 1995 experience in India when an explosive outbreak of plague occurred. Tetracycline was shown to be very effective and publicly demanded as the chosen mode of therapy. Actually, supplies

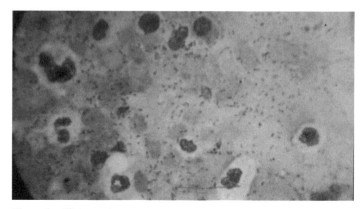

Plague bacilli (smear)

dwindled to a critical level, but the outbreak was brought under control.

REFERENCES

1. Woodward TE, Raby WT, Eppes E, Holbrook WA, Hightower JA. Aureomycin in the treatment of experimental and human tularemia. JAMA 1949;130:830–832.

2. Parker RT, Lister LM, Bauer RE, Hall HE, Woodward TE. Use of Chloromycetin in experimental and human tularemia. JAMA 1950; 143:7–11.

3. McCrumb FR, Snyder MJ, Woodward TE. Studies on human infection with *Pasteurella tularensis*. 1. Comparison of streptomycin and chloramphenicol in the prophylaxis of clinical disease. Trans Assoc Am Physicians 1947;70:74–79.

4. Smadel JE, Woodward TE, Amies CR, Goodner, K. Antibiotics in the treatment of bubonic and pneumonic plague in man. Ann NYork Acad Sci 1952;55:1275–1284.

5. McCrumb FR Jr, Mercier S, Robic J, Bouilat M, Smadel JE, Woodward TE, Goodner K. Chloramphenicol and terramycin in the treatment of pneumonic plague. Am J Med 1953;14:284–293.

6. Woodward TE, Petersdorf RG. The chemoprophylaxis of infection. II. The use of antibiotics to prevent infections by specific pathogens. J Pediatr 1961;58:153–163.

9

LEPTOSPIROSIS (WEIL'S DISEASE)

Theodore E. Woodward, M.D.

Our interests in leptospirosis (Weil's disease) were constantly stimulated by sporadic cases admitted to our medical wards or in local hospitals. St. Agnes Hospital was a particularly active site because of its location either near an abattoir or meat production plant. Febrile patients often went to St. Agnes whose medical staff kindly called us for consultation. Actually, we constantly kept several 400-gram guinea pigs on hand, useful for isolation of leptospires from the patients' blood or urine.

A particularly interesting patient of ours, in the late 1940s, was a severely ill young man who worked as a poultry plucker in a shop adjacent to the old Baltimore Harbor where cobblestone streets, Chesapeake Bay steamers, and rats helped make downtown memorable. The patient, who was first febrile, then severely jaundiced with a renal shutdown, fully recovered. Fortunately, we made a film sequence of the entire clinical picture which now serves for teaching purposes.

About this time when the undeclared war in Korea was brewing, we were attempting to reshape the Department of Med-

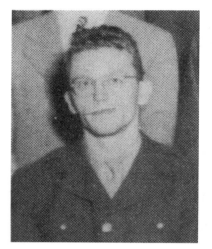

Howard E. Hall, M.D.

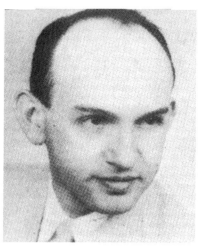

Kyle Y. Swisher, Jr., M.D.

icine at the University of Maryland School of Medicine in Baltimore. There were no state-
derived funds available for
medical research, even though
University President, H. Curley
Byrd, practically dominated the
Annapolis legislature in terms
of financial support for the
University. After the successful
venture in Kuala Lumpur in
Malaya, we had received a certain amount of much needed
confidence and recognition.

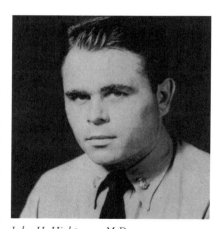

John H. Hightower, M.D.

During the early stages of the Korean Conflict, we had depth
in young, able physicians who were prepared and eager for challenges. Furthermore, the opportunity to be engaged in clinical
work in Puerto Rico had considerable more appeal than assignment to Korea! During their residency training, well-trained
young clinicians were taught the basics of laboratory support and
the means of confirming the specific diagnosis of infectious diseases. Our clinical research laboratory had a wide range of capability. Howard Hall, Kyle Swisher, and Jack Hightower were inducted into the U.S. Army as Captains in the Medical Corps with

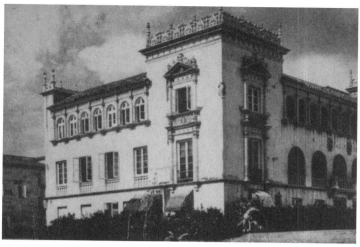

The School of Tropical Medicine, Puerto Rico

assignment for work at the Army Tropical Medicine Installation in San Juan, Puerto Rico. Funds derived from the McCormick Company were applied directly to support the laboratory unit there. These three physicians quickly gained permission to perform clinical work with public patients at the University Medical School Hospitals in San Juan. Simultaneously, a working relationship was developed with the correctional system in Puerto Rico permitting clinical studies to be conducted that were relevant to the health needs of inmates.

This clinical program in tropical medicine occurred at the same time as an insurrection, a prison outbreak, and an assassination attempt on the life of President Harry Truman while he addressed the Congress of the United States. Many Puerto Rican prisoners escaped and for several days wandered aimlessly in the environs of San Juan. They were hopelessly lost and soon wet with the brackish filthy water and mud in the poverty-stricken and congested ghettos. Once apprehended by insular authorities, they were returned to prison. An unusual febrile illness developed in many of the exposed victims. Hall, Swisher, and Hightower made the appropriate clinical observations, performed the necessary simple but important diagnostic tests, including strain isolation, and confirmed the strange illness as leptospirosis. Up to this time, leptospirosis or Weil's disease (severely ill, jaundiced cases) was regarded as rare in Puerto Rico and elsewhere in the Caribbean.[1-4]

U.S. Army Medical Officers, particularly Col. William (Bill) Gochenour (VMC), Col. Abram (Bud) Benenson (MC), and others from WRAIR, converged on Puerto Rico and soon confirmed the presence of the extensive epidemic. The clinical laboratory and epidemiologic studies showed that many heretofore unknown leptospiral strains were prevalent in Puerto Rico. There were many more confirmed cases without classic jaundice (yellow skin color) than those with jaundice. This was a new finding. Also, the various types of treatment that we utilized showed that antibiotics were not significantly helpful. These findings were contrary to earlier favorable reports.

My visit soon after the prison outbreak opened our eyes to the point that jaundice was uncommon in this illness and that splenomegaly was not a requirement for diagnosis. This work helped rewrite the medical chapters on this subject.[5-7] Kyle Swisher became a leading practicing cardiologist in Baltimore, first at the University of Maryland, and then at the St. Agnes Hospital. Jack Hightower, a very competent physician and internist, practiced medicine in Brunswick, Georgia. Howard Hall never left Maryland during his active practice career and became a leader in Carroll County and Sykesville. Bud Benenson is a recognized authority in epidemiology and infectious diseases, and Bill Gochenour became one of the leading veterinary officers in the U.S. Medical Corps.

In 1956, Fred McCrumb, while directing the WRAIR Program in Infectious Diseases in Kuala Lumpur, Malaya, made a comprehensive study of leptospirosis, particularly the type acquired during military operations in the jungle.[8] He and the group there showed that a type of leptospirosis with a short febrile course was a very common cause of obscure fever particularly in a tropical environment.[6,7] Its increased incidence was related to the time of exposure to brackish water. Earlier in 1955, Charley Wisseman, Bob Traub, and their associates reported a high incidence of leptospirosis in humans and animals in jungle areas of Southeast Asia.[9]

An interesting vignette demonstrated the ubiquity of leptospirosis. In the summer of 1942, about 40 cases of a febrile illness occurred in U.S. military troops stationed at Fort Bragg,

North Carolina. Dr. Worth Daniels and Dr. H.A. Grennan reported the unknown illness as Fort Bragg or pretibial fever. During the subsequent two summers , a similar number of cases occurred. The specific diagnosis was elusive for about 10 years, with dengue and a form of rickettsial disease as leading possibilities. Dr. Hugh Tatlock successfully isolated an agent by inoculating fertile hens' eggs with blood from patients. The unknown agent failed to kill the embryo and was successfully transferred from egg to egg and ultimately to hamsters. Hamsters failed to become seriously ill when inoculated with the unknown infected material.

In 1952, Joseph E. Smadel re-examined the records and febrile charts of some of the Fort Bragg cases in his laboratory at WRAIR. Jack Hightower also evaluated the febrile curves and clinical records. He remarked to Smadel, "in Puerto Rico, this would be called leptospirosis!" That was enough. Joe Smadel sent some of the previously stored Fort Bragg fever sera to Gochenour, at WRAIR, for testing with the various strains of leptospiras. When tested for *L. autumnalis* (a previously recognized Japanese strain) the titers went sky high. Previously, they had been tested for the three common strains: *L. ictero haemorrhagiae*, *L. canicola*, and *L. pomona*. There is little antigenic crossing among strains. Also, the hamsters, still in passage transfer of an agent, showed viable leptospiras on dark field examination of peritoneal exudate. Imagine the newspaper headlines in 1942; *Japanese Strain of Leptospirosis present in American Soldiers!*

REFERENCES

1. Hall HE, Hightower JA, Diaz-Rivera R, Bryne RJ, Smadel JE, Woodward TE. Evaluation of antibiotic therapy in human leptospirosis. Ann Intern Med 1951;35:981–998.

2. Woodward TE, Diaz-Rivera RS, Hightower JA. The variable clinical manifestations of leptospirosis. Bull NY Acad Med 1953;29: 642–647.

3. Stockard JL, Woodward TE. Leptospirosis: Infections in man. Vet Med 1957;52:548–552.

4. Diaz-Rivera RS, Ramos-Morales F, Benenson AF, Hall HE, Marchang EJ. Leptospiral meningitis. AMA Arch Intern Med 1959; 103:586–896.

5. Woodward TE, Hightower JA. The protean clinical features of leptospirosis. Maryland State Med J 1953;2:486–489.

6. McCrumb FR, Stockard JL, Woodward TE: Leptospirosis as a major cause of short term pyrexia in a tropical environment. Trans Assoc Am Phys 1956;69:122–130.

7. Stockard JL, Woodward TE. Leptospirosis: Infections in man. Ann NY Acad Sci 1958;70:414–420.

8. McCrumb FR Jr, Stockard JL, Robinson CR, Turner LH, Levis DG, Maisey CW, Kelleher MF, Gleiser CA, Smadel JE. Leptospirosis in Malaya. I. Sporadic cases among military and civilian personnel. Am J Trop Med Hyg 1957;6:238–256.

9. Wisseman CL Jr, Traub R, Gochenour WS Jr, Smadel JE, Lancaster WE. Leptospirosis of man and animals in urban, rural and jungle areas of Southeast Asia. J Trop Med Hyg 1955;4:29–40.

10

KOREAN HEMORRHAGIC FEVER

Theodore E. Woodward, M.D.

Korean hemorrhagic fever (KHF) became a tragic encounter beginning in 1952 when American troops were militarily engaged near the 38th Parallel. Not only were we ill-prepared for the events which followed, but the disease rates and high incidence of fatal cases were alarming as well as of significant strategic importance.

Many well-qualified and patriotic medical scientists such as Drs. William L. Jellison, W. Barry Wood, Jr., Robert Traub, Marshall Hertig, David Earle, and others had made fundamental observations directed toward helping clarify the hemorrhagic fever enigma.[1-7] In 1953, Joe Smadel, Scientific Director of the Walter Reed Army Institute of Research (WRAIR), decided on a direct approach and garnered Drs. Colin MacLeod, Adam Rapalski, Kenneth Goodner, Richard Mason, Thomas Wayne, and Ted Woodward for a fresh evaluation.

When arriving in Korea in September 1953, we became immediately involved in a difficult and most serious problem. Whenever young American soldiers contracted hemorrhagic fever and developed the shock syndrome, about 20% died in spite of

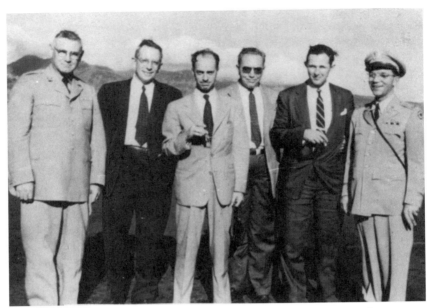

Korean Hemorrhagic Fever Mission: Tom Wayne, Joe Smadel, Colin MacLeod, John Dingle, Ted Woodward, and Adam Rapalski

any form of treatment. This death rate, for any illness, is unacceptable. By good fortune, one evening during a medical session, Col. Dick Mason sat next to Lt. Shelly Greisman and learned of his strong background, training, and experience in vascular physiology. He was an honor graduate of New York University School of Medicine in 1949 and a protégé of Drs. David Earle and Ludwig Eichna with whom he had worked on the capillary circulation. Joe Smadel and Dick Mason then arranged Greisman's transfer from the psychiatric service to which he had been assigned. Hemorrhagic fever, with its circulatory abnormalities, was just the kind of problem made for Greisman's expertise because it involved shock and an

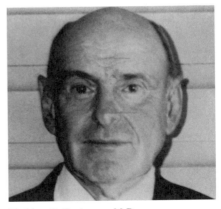

Sheldon E. Greisman, M.D.

understanding of the lesser circulation. His bedside observations and direct measurements of the capillary system led to significant clarification, proving to be an important addition of new knowledge of this strange illness. Greisman's studies revealed a biphasic response of the capillary beds with dilatation and hyporesponsiveness to catecholamines and very sensitive hyperreactivity of the capillary circulation to catecholamines. This correlated with the hypotensive and hypertensive phases of illness and appeared to explain the gross alterations in cardiovascular dynamics.

George Entwisle, a Tufts Medical School product and a former trainee under Dr. Chester Keefer, was hard at work as a medical officer in a forward 48th M.A.S.H. unit. Many soldiers with hemorrhagic fever were hospitalized there, having been transported to the medical unit by helicopter. Administration of excess fluids, intravenously, during the period of early shock and renal shutdown invariably caused subsequent marked edema of the lungs, brain, and subcutaneous tissues— and often death. Entwisle, Greisman, and the group showed that very limited infusions of fluid given intravenously with small titrated doses of epinephrine to barely maintain the blood pressure and cerebral and renal circulation were effective. This clinical work was a critical step in helping salvage these seriously ill young men.

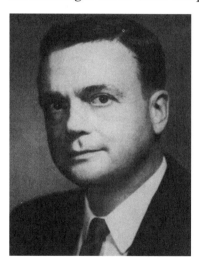

George Entwistle, M.D.

The medical profession was to hear more about the hemorrhagic fevers later with Lassa fever, Marburg virus infection, Bolivian hemorrhagic fever, and the hantavirus.

A training film was made of KHF by the Photographic Division of WRAIR. It vividly displays the clinical manifestations, pathophysiologic abnormalities, pathologic findings, and laboratory diagnostic aids. It is available in the WRAIR, Armed Forces Institute of Pathology (AFIP), and University of Maryland film collection.

After the Korean conflict, Greisman and Entwisle accepted the invitation to leave New York and Boston, respectively, and join our Department of Medicine in Baltimore. Working with the Infectious Diseases Division, Greisman developed into one of the country's leading authorities in the field of bacterial endotoxins and clinical physiology.

Entwisle engaged in clinical practice on a geographical full-time basis, directed the large medical outpatient clinic, and ultimately succeeded Dr. Pincoffs as Head of the Department of Preventive Medicine and Rehabilitation in 1958.

This same medical trip enabled me to meet Capt. William S. Spicer, a University of Kansas medical graduate (1949) who was busy with an Infantry Unit at the 38th parallel in Korea. After the war, Spicer joined our department, headed our Division of Pulmonary Medicine, and developed much new knowledge on the relationship of environmental pollution and chronic lung disease. Later, his innovative Primary Care Training Program, which included clinical units with nurses, pharmacists, and allied health personnel, became a model health care system.

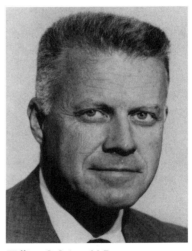

William S. Spicer, M.D.

When our military forces were first exposed to and contracted Korean hemorrhagic fever in 1950, there were many gaps in the available information. Of particular importance was the animal reservoir, if any, and the mode of transmission of the agent to humans, such as an ectoparasite. Through their epidemiologic studies in Korea, Traub, Wisseman, and collaborators correctly predicted that the virus of KHF was prevalent in North American rodents.[7,8] Of more striking significance was the team contribution which led to the first isolation of Congo-Crimean hemorrhagic fever virus from ticks in 1970.[9] The work on tick-borne viruses was conducted under the International Center for Medical Research and Training (ICMRT) Program in Pakistan.

REFERENCES

1. Giles RB, Sheedy JA, Ekman CN, Froeb HE, Conley CC, Stockard JL, Cugeil DW, Vester JW, Kiyasu RK, Entwisle G, Yoe RH. The sequelae of epidemic hemorrhagic fever. Am J Med 1954;16:629.

2. Sayer WJ, Entwisle G, Uyeno B, Bignall RC. Cortisone therapy of early hemorrhagic fever: a preliminary report. Ann Intern Med 1955; 42:839.

3. Greisman S.E. The reactivity of the capillary bed of the nail fold to circulating epinephrine and norepinephrine in patients with normal blood pressure and with essential hypertension. J Clin Invest 1952;31: 782.

4. Greisman S.E. The reaction of the capillary bed of the nail fold to the continuous intravenous infusion of levo-norepinephrine in patients with normal blood pressure and with essential hypertension. J Clin Invest 1954;33:975.

5. Greisman S.E. The regulation of effective circulating blood volume. Med Bull U.S. Army 1954;2:32.

6. Greisman SE. Capillary observations in patients with hemorrhagic fever and other infectious illnesses. J Clin Invest 1957;36:1688

7. Traub R, Wisseman CL Jr. Editorial: Korean hemorragic fever. J Infect Dis 1978;138(2):267–272.

8. Lee PW, Yanagihara R, Franko RC, Amyx HL, Gibbs CJ Jr, Gajdusek DC, Traub R. Letter to the Editor concerning Korean hemorrhagic fever infection in rodents. N Engl J Med 1982;307(10):624–625.

9. Begum F, Wisseman CL Jr, Traub R. Tick-borne viruses of West Pakistan. I. Isolation and general characteristics. Am J Epidemiol 1970; 92(3):180–191.

11

Asiatic Cholera

Theodore E. Woodward, M.D.

Cholera has ravaged the Asian subcontinent for centuries, always present in India and East Pakistan (Bangladesh) with a heavy toll in numbers of cases and deaths. It has periodically spread to adjacent countries and elsewhere. This occurred in Thailand, Hong Kong, the Philippines, and throughout the Far East, beginning in 1958. Western Europe and North and South America have been periodically involved with epidemic cholera.

BASIC STUDIES

During 1959, a combined team consisting of scientists from the Walter Reed Army Institute of Research (WRAIR) and the National Institutes of Health (NIH) worked collaboratively in Bangkok, Thailand, with a U.S. Navy research team, Thai investigators, epidemiologists, and allied health personnel. Dr. Eugene Gangarosa, who later joined the Division of Infectious Diseases, performed key studies in pathophysiology of cholera while in Bangkok.[1]

In 1959, Dr. James H. Shannon, Director of NIH, was requested by the Department of State to suggest and develop a health program to help people of Southeast Asia under the auspices of the South East Asia Treaty Organization (SEATO). Dr. Shannon asked his deputy director, Dr. Joseph E. Smadel, to develop a program with starting funds in the amount of $400,000 derived from the International Cooperative Administration (ICA). Smadel convened a small working group consisting of Kenneth Goodner (Jefferson), John H. Dingle (Case Western Reserve), Colin M. Macleod (Pennsylvania), Richard Mason (WRAIR), and Theodore E. Woodward (Maryland). In their monograph on "The American Scientific Experience on Cholera, 1947–1980," Van Heyningen and Seal spoke of this group as an "Inner Circle" consisting of a few in the upper management of science who were old enough still to be interested in tropical diseases despite the trend away from them.[2]

Asiatic cholera then afflicted South Asian people and caused unprecedented deaths and morbidity. In order to assess the magnitude of the problem and develop a better understanding of the facts, known and unknown about the threat, the group visited leading centers in the Far East. A series of conferences and workshops were held at the National Institutes of Health, Tokyo and the Kitasato Institute. Taipei proved to be the most important site visit because Capt. Robert Phillips, USN, Commandant of the Navy Research Unit (NAMRU-2), and his staff were conducting landmark physiologic studies of the various abnormalities in cholera, and therapy based on fluid replacement. Much helpful information was gleaned in Taipei regarding diagnosis, pathogenesis, and control of cholera.

Manila, Hong Kong, New Delhi, and Calcutta were visited. Neither the Philippines nor Hong Kong seemed appropriate for establishing a cholera study center because the disease was not endemically planted there.

The reception of the team in Bangkok was vigorous and affable. The relationship with the military services and academic centers all looked promising. The problem was simply that cholera outbreaks in Thailand were sporadic, making contact with human cases difficult.

Although cholera was rampant in India, particularly in Calcutta, a study center was precluded because India was not a member nation of SEATO. Many world authorities on cholera worked in India's various medical centers, including the Health Ministry in Delhi.

In Dacca, East Pakistan, everything was ideal for placement of a cholera research laboratory. Cholera patients were accessible every year in large numbers. The disease was permanently established in this population-dense country, which during wet seasons was partially inundated by flood waters. Public health standards were poor, and authorities were anxious and enthusiastic for a research center there. An entire wing of the Public Health Institute was available for laboratory space, clinical studies, and administration. Here the SEATO Cholera Research Center found a permanent home.[3]

A second center under U.S. Department of Defense (WRAIR) auspices, including a working affiliation, was recommended for Bangkok. In presenting its recommendations, the group felt that the site visits had been productive, and the outcome would prove successful.

The Dacca Center ultimately developed into the leading cholera laboratory and clinical investigative unit in the world. It functioned under a special advisory group of NIH Bethesda, and soon profited from international participation by scientists from England, France, Australia, Pakistan, and the United States. It became the site for young clinical investigators with physiologic

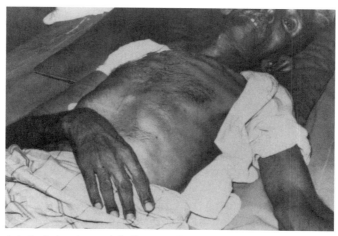

Asiatic cholera in an adult (Courtesy SEATO Cholera Research Laboratory)

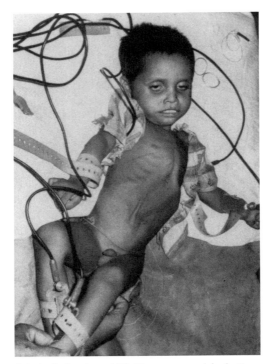

Asiatic cholera in a child. Note extreme dehydration.
(Courtesy SEATO Cholera Research Laboratory)

and immunologic interests to contribute importantly, grow academically, and ultimately take key positions elsewhere.

From Maryland, many young physicians trained and contributed. These included Drs. Richard Cash, Robert Gilman, Stanley Music, David Nalin, Merrill Snyder, Richard Wenzel, and William E. Woodward. Numerous visits were made by Dr. Richard Hornick, as well as Dr. T.E. Woodward, who served on the NIH Advisory Committee.

ORAL REHYDRATION

In December 1960, following the SEATO Conference on cholera in Dacca, Woodward served as rapporteur for the section on clinical manifestation and management. Dr. Smadel assigned each rapporteur the responsibility to propose future "Directions of the Wind" based on proposed needs. Woodward's comments follow[3]:

Woodward

> Dehydrated patients are thirsty. Cholera patients are no exception, although vomiting interferes with administering fluids via the natural route. No effective means other than intravenous alimentation has allayed this sign. Perhaps an efficient antiemetic medication or other means would serve a useful role and aid those patients for whom intravenous fluids are unavailable. (pp. 324–325)

Woodward also proposed:

> Should antibacterial drugs be given a critical trial before they are scrapped from the cholera regimen? The study should be designed carefully, using sufficient numbers of patients who receive antibacterial drugs and appropriate fluid and electrolyte replacement and a control group who receive only the replacement therapy. Whether the sulfonamides, antibiotics or steroids are useful or necessary is unknown since there are no reliable control data.

As later shown, oral replacement alimentation became dramatically effective.[3–10] This represented a major contribution for treatment of the serious dehydrating diarrheal diseases.

THERAPY

Tetracycline, reported by the Hopkins ICMRT group in Calcutta and the SEATO Lab group in Dacca, effectively reduced the requirement for fluid replacement and cut, by half, the shedding of *Vibrio. cholerae* in the stool.[11]

These associations, and Division interests, involving work on enteric diseases, as well as the need to develop new knowledge about vaccines, prompted the study of cholera in volunteers. Such work was vital in order to assess and fully appraise the efficacy of cholera vaccines in field trials. There were controversial questions concerning 1) the effectiveness of cholera toxoid, 2) the importance of antitoxic or antibacterial immunity, 3) the relative importance of coproantibody or intestinal lumen immunity, and 4) the future promise of living or molecularly manipulated cholera vaccines. These issues were addressed in the enteric diseases study (typhoid fever, bacillary dysentery, and *E. coli* diarrhea) (see later sections).

The initial requirement in order to obtain answers to the potential objectives was to determine the infectious dose of *V. cholerae* for humans. There was sufficient capability and confidence that an induced infection in humans could be promptly and adequately managed. These cholera volunteer studies, in 1970–1971, were directed by Dr. Hornick.[12]

Oral vaccines seemed to be feasible for typhoid fever and cholera, based on the ongoing studies. Later, live attenuated vaccine strains of specific bacteria were given to volunteers who were subsequently challenged with pathogenic strains. Manipulated vaccine strains not only conferred protection against developing clinical manifestations, but shortened the time of shedding typhoid or cholera organisms in the stools.[13–15]

Dr. Myron Levine took over responsibility for the volunteer program in 1974. In 1983, the unit was formally designated as a separate division, The Center for Vaccine Development. A one-dose live cholera vaccine, genetically engineered, was later developed and tested in a large-scale field trial in Indonesia.[16,17] It showed remarkably good results and is now licensed.

A one-dose live oral typhoid vaccine was evaluated in Phase 2 clinical studies in university student volunteers. Ultimately, Phase 3 trials were performed in South America all under WHO, the Research and Development Command of the Department of Defense, and NIH sponsorship and support. Results were favorable and gratifying when compared with other available vaccines.

RELATED CONTRIBUTIONS

Dr. Albert T. Dawkins (Skip) and Dr. Stanley (Stan) Music were equally effective in evaluating such enteric infections. Skip Dawkins's work carried over to critical evaluation of vaccine efficacy in Rocky Mountain spotted fever. These pioneering studies involved identification of virulence factors and control with inactivated and viable vaccines given orally. All of this work included carefully controlled trials of protective efficacy in humans. These team contributions helped place the infectious disease program on a solid and effective foundation.

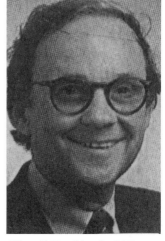

Albert T. Dawkins, Jr., M.D.

A particularly innovative contribution was made by John C. Harris, a medical student who, with Bert Dupont, showed for the first time that the use of methylene blue greatly simplified the identification of leukocytes in fecal smears. This technique ultimately became a standard practice.

Ronica Kluge came as a house officer in medicine from the University of Florida and then trained with us as a fellow in infectious diseases in 1971. She served as an important member of our faculty until 1974. In addition to her most effective teaching talents, she investigated important and innovative problems related to superimposed infections, their pathogenesis, and means of control. She studied antibiotic combinations and pinpointed important abnormalities in patients with bacteremia which led to mortality. Later, she served as a faculty member in infectious diseases at the University of West Virginia Medical School and the University of Texas Medical School, Galveston, before settling for medical practice at the Southwest Florida Regional Medical Center, Ft. Myers.

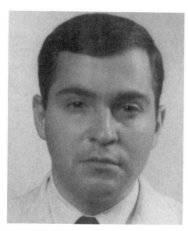

Joseph P. Libonati, Ph.D.
Asst. Prof. Medicine

Dr. Joseph P. Libonati who held joint appointments in microbiology and medicine (infectious diseases) contributed importantly to studies on pathogenesis and control of bacillary dysentery and typhoid fever. Later, he became Chief, Division of Microbiology and Deputy Director, Laboratory Administration, Maryland Department of Health and Mental Hygiene.

REFERENCES

1. Gangarosa EJ, Beisel WR, Benyayati C, Sprinz H, Piyaratn P. The nature of the gastrointestinal lesion in Asiatic cholera and its relation to pathogenesis: a biopsy study. Am J Trop Med Hyg 1960;9:125.

2. Van Heyningen WE, Seal Jr. Cholera, The American Scientific Experience 1947–1980. Westview Press: Boulder, CO, 1983.

3. SEATO Conference on Cholera. Public Health Rep 1961;76: 323.

4. Nalin DR. Sucrose in oral therapy for cholera and related diarrheas. Lancet 1975;1:1400.

5. Nalin DR, Cash RA. Oral or nasogastric maintenance therapy for diarrhea of unknown etiology resembling cholera. Trans R Soc Trop Med Hyg 1970;64:769.

6. Nalin DR, Cash RA. Oral or nastrogastric maintenance therapy in pediatric cholera patients. J Pediatr 1971;78:355.

7. Nalin DR, Cash RA, Islam R, Motta M, Phillips RA. Oral maintenance therapy for cholera in adults. Lancet 1968;2:370.

8. Nalin DR, Cash RA, Rahman M. Oral (or nasogastric) maintenance therapy for cholera patients in all age-groups. Bull WHO 1970;43:361.

9. Nalin DR, Cash RA, Rahman M, Ynus M. Effect of glycine and glucose on sodium and water absorption in patients with cholera. Gut 1970;11:768.

10. Nalin DR, Levine MM, Hornick RB, Berquist EJ, Hoover D, Holley HP, Waterman D, Van Blerk J, Matheney S, Sotman S, Rennels M. The problem of emesis during oral glucose-electrolyte therapy given from the onset of severe cholera. Trans R Soc Trop Med Hyg, 1978;13:10.

11. Greenough WB III, Gordon RS, Rosenberg IS, Davies BI, Benenson AS. Tetracycline in the treatment of cholera. Lancet 1964;1:355.

12. Hornick RB, Music SE, Wenzel R, Cash R, Libonati JP, Snyder MJ, Woodward TE. The Broad Street pump revisited: Response of volunteers to ingested cholera vibrio. NY Acad Bull 1971;46:(10):1181–1971.

13. Hornick RB, DuPont HL, Levine MM, Gilman RH, Woodward WE, Snyder MJ, Woodward TE. Efficacy of a live oral typhoid vaccine in human volunteers. Dev Biol Stand 1955;33:89–92.

14. Gilman RH, Hornick RB, Woodward WE, DuPont HL, Snyder MJ, Levine MM, Liboneti JF. Evaluation of a VDP glucose-4 epimeraseless mutant of salmonella typhi as a live oral vaccine. J Infect Dis 1977;136:717–723.

15. Tacket CO, Hone DM, Losonsky GA, Guera L, Edelman R, Levine MM. Clinical acceptability and immunogenicity of CVD 908 salmonella typhi vaccine strain. Vaccine 1992;10(7):443–446.

16. Woodward WE, Gilman RH, Hornick RB, Libonati JP, Cash RA. Efficacy of a live oral-cholera vaccine in human volunteers. Fourteenth Congress of the International Association of Biological Standardization, Douglas, Isle of Man, 1975. Dev Biol Stand 1976;33:108–112.

17. Levine MM, Kaper JB, Herrington D, Ketley J, Losonsky G, Tacket CO, Tall B, Cryz S. Safety, immunogenicity and efficacy of recombinant live oral cholera vaccines. CVD 103 and CVD 103, HgR. Lancet 1988;27:467–470.

12

TRAINING, RESEARCH, AND COMMUNITY-ORIENTED MEDICINE 1954–1958

Robert T. Parker, M.D.

My fellowship in infectious diseases began on July 1, 1949, as the successor to Dr. William Holbrook. Dr. Woodward introduced me to Leonard Lister, a senior medical student, who took me to the section's laboratory, consisting of two small rooms and an animal room on the fifth floor of the Bressler Research Building. Division personnel at the time were Ann Meredith, a full-time technician, and Dr. Fred Mc-Crumb, a medical house officer, who dedicated many hours to research for this section. Carol Young was the devoted Division secretary. During the summer months, we

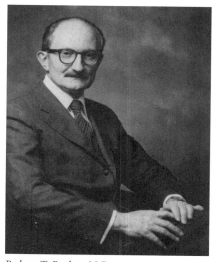

Robert T. Parker, M.D.

107

made rounds in the hospital, keeping detailed records and collecting specimens from patients with Rocky Mountain spotted fever, typhoid fever, aseptic meningitis, brucellosis, tuberculous meningitis, pneumonia, and tularemia. In addition, I went to Fort Howard, Mercy, and St. Joseph Hospitals providing medical consultations and obtaining detailed patient information later used in publications, such as the first and second reports of chloramphenicol treatment for Rocky Mountain spotted fever.[1,2]

Our efforts at isolating pathogenic rickettsiae were limited to injecting the patient's blood intraperitoneally into guinea pigs, taking daily temperatures, and, at an appropriate time, sacrificing the animal for attempted transfer of the agent to fertile hens' eggs. A new experience was to candle eggs in order to identify fertile ones!

Although we were at some risk in handling such rickettsial pathogens in the laboratory, the experience with *Pasteurella tularensis* was another matter! During those early days, Ann Meredith and Leonard Lister each contracted severe tularemia involving the lungs. There were no protective hoods, and the procedure of pipetting infectious material from tube to tube could be hazardous.

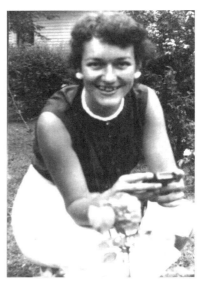

Ann Meredith, Ph.D.

With regard to the risk of contracting tularemia and contamination, Dr. Woodward was invited to give lectures to second-year microbiology students at Johns Hopkins Medical School. Our technician prepared the *P. tularensis* cultures on chocolate agar slants and took the cultures to Hopkins. Because of the highly infectious characteristics of these organisms, she was met with considerable apprehension. Considerable caution was taken in transfer of cultures and staining procedures. Upon completion of Woodward's lecture on tularemia, the slant cultures were distributed to the students for the practice exercises. One bright young student called Dr. Woodward for examination of his microscopic specimen because he identified the microorganism as staphylococcus. Much to his chagrin, Dr. Woodward had to agree!

After the summer period and with the onset of the scholastic year, Leonard Lister returned to his medical studies. Dr. McCrumb continued his work in evaluating the efficacy of chloramphenicol and Aureomycin in treatment of pneumococcal, meningococcal, and *Hemophilus influenzae* meningitis. In October, Dr. Howard Hall joined the section as part of his internal medicine University Hospital residency. Next came Dr. Merrill Snyder, recruited by Dr. Woodward from the Walter Reed Medical Center. Merrill's serologic and bacteriologic expertise greatly expanded our capabilities. In November, Dr. Woodward received a request from Drs. William Lowe and Rodney Layton to come to investigate an outbreak of "virus pneumonia" in Queenstown, Easton, and surrounding sections of the Eastern Shore. Initially, Drs. Woodward, Hall, and Parker responded and visited many homes of ill persons. Subsequently, Snyder, Hall, and I were ferried across the Chesapeake Bay many times to visit patients, obtain accurate historical data, collect sputum and blood specimens, and distribute chloramphenicol and Aureomycin. These visits were regular and routine. We became familiar and friendly with many Eastern Shoremen. On one occasion, we were reported to be Bible salesmen! The serologic specimens we collected were tested for the presence of antibodies and specific agents of brucellosis, tularemia, Q fever, and other pathogens. Ultimately, the outbreak was thought to be caused by mycoplasma pneumonia which had masqueraded as "atypical pneumonia."

In the Spring of 1950, the Division's overseas program in infectious diseases was formalized under Dr. Woodward's direction. Drs. Howard Hall, John Hightower, and Kyle Swisher, under U.S. Army auspices, were assigned to its Tropical Disease Laboratory in Puerto Rico. Here meningitis, typhoid fever, dysentery, and leptosporosis were intensively studied clinically and in the laboratory. Dr. Fred McCrumb first received special training on plague and went to Madagascar for evaluation of pneumonic plague. In Baltimore, the Division regularly accepted medical residents for three-month assignments from the University, Church Home, and Mercy Hospitals. Fellowship training funds were obtained for an organized training program, which included Drs. Joseph Workman, John Benson, Ray Liu, and others mentioned elsewhere.

During the early years, financial support for the Division was meager. Thanks to Dr. Woodward's tireless efforts, the section received grant support and generous supplies of antibiotics from the Lederle and Parke-Davis Corporations. Later, Dr. Gladys Hobby of Pfizer approached Dr. Woodward and requested that clinical trials be conducted with an Aureomycin derivative; we were delighted with this opportunity. Additionally, Mr. Charles P. McCormick contributed three successive annual grants of $10,000 each from the McCormick Company. Dr. Woodward had assisted in his medical care.

A far-reaching contribution of our Division's educational and research program was the active participation and involvement of faculty members and fellows in the study of infectious disease problems throughout Baltimore and Maryland. Their visits at all hours to hospitals and clinics on the Western and Eastern Shore sections of the state established an identity in infectious diseases for the Maryland Medical Center. Subsequently, this led to referrals of interesting and seriously ill patients, so necessary for successful conduct of meaningful research and comprehensive medical care. All of these efforts resulted in a recognized training program.

Not only was Dr. Woodward interested in acquiring grant support, but he never overlooked any opportunity, however small, to increase the Division's coffers. He conceived and put into operation a plan to place a soda-dispensing machine on our floor in Bressler so that the Division could receive a percentage of the sales. The machine was kept busy with active use by our personnel, as well as RH laboratory staff members. Our leader was a regular user, often crossing Greene Street to escape the teaching, administrative, and practice responsibilities, to take his lunch (a soda) and offer help and guidance.

A very significant event occurred as a result of one of these visits. Dr. Woodward always taught Zinsser's hypothesis, that patients with rickettsial diseases, who survived, usually had viable rickettsia latent in their reticulo-endothelial systems. Clinically, Zinsser had identified recurrent typhus fever or Brill's disease as the best example. However, the existence of such symbiosis had not been proven.

In 1949, a patient gravely ill with Rocky Mountain spotted fever was treated at University Hospital with chloramphenicol and fortunately survived. Eighteen months later, Dr. Woodward persuaded the patient to submit for excision of an inguinal lymph node. After being brought to the Division's laboratory, one half of the node was frozen, and the other half was given to our personnel with instructions to attempt rickettsiae isolation, first by inoculation of guinea pigs and later to fertile hens' eggs. Our attempt resulted in failure.

On one of the above mentioned "Coke" visits, Dr. Woodward personally ground up the remaining one half of the lymph node and injected it into guinea pigs. The guinea pigs were also given large doses of corticosteroids. He took daily rectal temperatures of the animals, sacrificed them at the appropriate time, and transferred the necessary tissue specimens into fertile hens' eggs. Subsequently, viable rickettsiae were isolated. Dr. Snyder then performed the necessary serologic tests to confirm isolation of the "Matthews strain" of microorganisms taken 18 months after the patient's recovery from a near-fatal disease. This first written confirmation of a long suspected relationship of microbial persistence was prepared for publication by the principal investigator and assigned to me for presentation at the American Federation of Clinical Research's annual meeting. This permitted my election to membership in the Federation, an honor which I cherish.

Several years later, the same technical procedure was employed by Dr. Winston Price at Hopkins and Dr. Joseph Smadel's team in Malaysia, confirming the same host–parasite relationship for epidemic and scrub typhus fevers.

Throughout the years, the Division's activities included research projects, publications, teaching, and training, all spearheaded by Dr. Woodward. Dr. Merrill Snyder performed an extensive serologic survey of cattle and sheep in Maryland searching for an accurate incidence of Q fever. These classic findings were used for his doctoral thesis. Dr. Shelley Greisman reported broadly on his important microvascular studies, including the effects of endotoxins. Dr. Joseph Workman collected basic clinical data which showed that cortisone in conjunction with antibiotics assisted in treatment of Rocky Mountain spotted fever (RMSF) and other infectious diseases. Many projects initiated by Dr. Woodward expanded greatly after 1958 when I resigned the Directorship to be succeeded by Dr. Fred McCrumb.

From 1954 to 1958, the Division contributed importantly to the broad-spectrum antibiotic treatment of tularemia and purulent meningitis (1955). It was shown that chloramphenicol (Chloromycetin) had a wide spectrum of efficacy for the common types of meningitis (*H. influenzae*, pneumococcus, and meningococcus), with favorable action against other types. This antibiotic was shown to diffuse well to the meninges, cerebrospinal fluid, and subarachnoid space.

Another landmark publication (1954) was the report that *R. Rickettsii*, the agent which causes RMSF, persisted viably in lymphoid tissues for fully a year in convalescent patients. This confirmed Zinsser's older concept of microbial persistence to explain recurrent typhus fever (Brill-Zinsser disease). (See references in special sections on tularemia, meningitis, and rickettsial diseases).

REFERENCES

1. Pincoffs MC, Guy EG, Lister LM, Woodward TE, Smadel JE. The treatment of rocky mountain spotted fever with chloromycetin. Ann Intern Med 1949;209:656–663.

2. Parker RT, Bauer RE, Lister LM, Woodward TE, Hall HE. Further experience in the treatment of rocky mountain spotted fever with chloramphenicol. Am J Med 1950;9:308–314.

13

THE EFFECT OF TOXINS, PEPTIDES, AND IMMUNE REACTIONS ON PATHOGENESIS, TREATMENT, AND CONTROL OF RICKETTSIAL DISEASES, TYPHOID FEVER, HEMORRHAGIC FEVER, AND GRAM-NEGATIVE SEPSIS

Sheldon E. Greisman, M.D.

KOREAN EPIDEMIC HEMORRHAGIC FEVER

My first glimpse of Ted Woodward occurred at a 38th Parallel Medical Conference in Korea in 1953. After having been initially assigned to be the 8th Army Division psychiatrist, I had been reassigned to the 48th M.A.S.H. (thanks to efforts of Col. Richard (Dick) Mason and Dr. Joseph (Joe) Smadel which overcame severe protests by the area psychiatric commandant). The new mission was to explore the microcirculatory derangements during Korean epidemic hemorrhagic fever (EHF). On this day, all

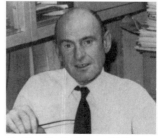

Sheldon E. Greisman, M.D.
Professor, Medicine, Physiology

medical personnel in the area had been "requested" (i.e., or-
dered) to attend a special medical conference, since a world famous physician was going to speak about rickettsial diseases.
The road was dusty, and the open jeep ride took about one hour.
We finally arrived at a large steel Quonset hut, filled to capacity
with several hundred medical officers seated on wooden folding
chairs. On the raised platform were a number of colonels and Joe
Smadel, dressed in army fatigues. He called for silence, the room
hushed, and Smadel introduced the famous speaker we had all
assembled to hear, Dr. Theodore E. Woodward, from the University of Maryland School of Medicine. The talk was entitled "You
Have to Pay the Piper," and the concept presented was that immunity to rickettsial disease could not be acquired simply by administering antibiotics during the incubation period; rather, periods of illness were needed to stimulate specific immunity in order
for early antibiotic therapy to be successful. It was a fascinating
talk and little did I realize then as Woodward was delivering his
speech dressed in combat boots and army fatigues that my life
shortly thereafter would be totally altered and molded by this
man who was to become the next Chairman of the Department
of Medicine at the University of Maryland School of Medicine,
as well as my subsequent lifelong friend.

At that time in Korea (1953), it had already become apparent that the major pathophysiologic derangements in EHF
resided in profound alterations in the microcirculatory system.
We observed that during the hypotensive phase of illness, the
capillary beds in the nailfold of the skin and conjunctivae became
markedly dilated, hyporesponsive to intravenous infusions of catecholamines, and exhibited increased permeability as evidenced
by areas of interstitial edema and extravasations of red blood
cells. Several days later, the microcirculation began to change
dramatically, becoming constricted, hyperresponsive to cate-
cholamine infusions, and the edema resorbed. Arterial blood
pressure which had decreased earlier now became elevated into
hypertensive ranges. Whatever the etiologic agent, it appeared to
be acting as a microvascular toxin, and we now sought to prove
its existence and then identify this toxin by transfer studies into
experimental animals.[1] Dr. Gordon Moe, Chairman of the Department of Pharmacology at the University of Syracuse School
of Medicine, initially assisted with these studies, and we were

able to demonstrate a microcirculatory vasodilator factor in serum of soldiers during the acute febrile and hypotensive phases of EHF. Based on these findings, Charles L. Wisseman was dispatched from the Walter Reed Army Institute of Research (WRAIR) to help isolate this vasodilator serum factor. We spent many months at the 48th M.A.S.H. tracking this factor and continued this work after returning to the United States where Dr. Wisseman became Chairman of the Department of Microbiology at the University of Maryland School of Medicine. It was at the invitation of Ted Woodward and Charles Wisseman that I received a joint one-year trial appointment in medicine and microbiology to continue these studies. We finally did identify the vasodilator factor. It turned out not to be a toxin, but rather was related to a complex interplay of several mechanisms, including heterophile agglutinins in human plasma in the animals with which we were working, rabbits and rats. When human plasma became rich in fatty acids, such as occurs during lipolysis after 48 hours of starvation, the interplay of these heterophile agglutinins, human complement, and fatty acids injured the experimental animal's erythrocytes sufficiently to release their high content of adenosine derivatives, which are potent microcirculatory vasodilators. We could reproduce the EHF "toxin" simply by fasting healthy volunteers until ketones appeared in their urine or, conversely, by feeding a high-fat diet to these volunteers. (On many occasions, Dr. Merrill Snyder volunteered to eat a pint of cream for these latter studies, but declined the former.) While disappointing, these data will be useful to future investigators attempting to demonstrate and isolate vaso-injurious factors in human plasma. Despite the disappointing results, my contract was renewed. Incidentally, the observations on the importance of fatty acids for liberation of vasodilatory adenosine derivates from erythrocytes led to a series of published studies detailing an interesting mechanism by which plasma proteins can either protect against or enhance the lysis of red blood cells by fatty acids.

ROLE OF LIPOPOLYSACCHARIDES

Since Charles Wisseman was particularly interested in the effects of rickettsial toxins on the microcirculation, we studied the effect of murine typhus on the microcirculation of the meso-appendix of the rat. We showed that these effects were quite distinct from those produced by Gram-negative bacterial endotoxin, lipopolysaccharide (LPS). Photographs of the alterations in the microcirculation induced by murine typhus and by LPS were published in conjunction with the details of these studies. Incidentally, during one of the experiments, a syringe loaded with "hot" murine typhus rickettsiae broke and sprayed the area under the primitive hood where we were working. Wisseman had been immunized and remained well, but one week later, as expected, my bout with murine typhus began. I refused antibiotics because of severe penicillin anaphylactic shock one year previously. Recovery began only after two weeks of a most debilitating febrile illness (headache was the most devastating symptom), during which Ted Woodward presented me before the entire sophomore class and after which Charles Wisseman (under orders from Joe Smadel) bled me repeatedly to obtain the highest titered anti-rickettsial antisera they had ever encountered. Woodward assures me that I still harbor the murine rickettsiae and speculates that some of the mild febrile illnesses since that time might represent the murine typhus equivalent of Brill-Zinnser illness.

Hemorrhagic Shock

My interest in endotoxin (LPS) began with the initial reports by Jacob Fine, a Harvard surgeon, that hemorrhagic shock becomes irreversible with time because of the collapse of the endotoxin detoxifying capacity of the reticuloendothelial system (RES). Endotoxins absorbed from the gut then produce the irreversible phase wherein restoration of blood volume no longer results in survival. Studies in our laboratory were begun to test this interesting hypothesis. Rabbits were bled into a reservoir until their mean arterial blood pressure reached levels that, if untreated for more than two hours, resulted in irreversibility, despite return of all shed blood. At two hours, when reversibility was still possible, blood was returned and the animals were titrated for sensitivity to intravenously injected LPS. We found that sensitivity to LPS did increase after such hemorrhage, but only modestly (100-fold), not by the 100,000-fold figure reported by Dr. Fine. Moreover, this modest increase in sensitivity could be correlated with growth of clostridia which are normally present in latent form in rabbit muscles and which were activated by the muscle dissection during cannulation of the femoral artery. Ligation of this major artery after return of the blood loss caused marked edema of the lower limb (assessed by postmortem weighing of the isolated extremity) and completed the setting for activation of the clostridial sepsis. Use of prophylactic local antibiotics in the area of the femoral cutdown, or clostridial antitoxin, or use of bleedouts by sterile cardiac puncture, markedly blunted or abolished the otherwise modest increases in sensitivity to LPS.[2]

Following these studies, our interest in LPS continued, since the possibility still remained unproven that irreversible hemorrhagic shock might be caused by gut-absorbed LPS, and since increased numbers of patients were being seen with Gram-negative bacterial (GNB) sepsis and septic shock. The focus now centered on the role of LPS in these syndromes and how the effect of LPS, if this was indeed a factor, could be neutralized. Initial studies to answer the latter question were concerned with the phenomenon of tolerance, wherein exposure to small amounts of LPS rapidly leads to remarkable increases in resistance to this toxin. The accepted hypothesis at that time had been proposed by Paul Beeson at Yale University School of Medicine. He postulated that the RES was stimulated by the initial injection of LPS so that subsequent injections were cleared more rapidly from the circulation, thereby diverting the LPS from the vulnerable target sites. This theory rested heavily upon the observation that "blockade" of the RES with colloids such as thorotrast slowed the intravascular clearance of LPS and abolished tolerance. We were the first to demonstrate that Beeson's theory was not tenable. Blockade of the RES with thorotrast was shown not to abolish tolerance, but rather simply to reset resistance to LPS at a lower level within the framework of the tolerant state; nontolerant animals given thorotrast became significantly more reactive to LPS than did tolerant animals given thorotrast, and this difference remained comparable to that observed in the absence of thorotrast.[3] These observations were later confirmed by other investigators. (After a talk given by Paul Beeson on eosinophils several decades later at The Johns Hopkins School of Medicine, I had the privilege of meeting Paul Beeson personally. I was both flattered and embarrassed by his unforgettable remark: "It is a pleasure to meet you. If I had known you were in the audience, I would have been more careful with the data.") Subsequently, it was shown by Elisha

Atkins at Yale, using in vitro techniques, and then in vivo by our laboratory, using perfusion of the portal vein of rabbits, that the RES was actually the major target of LPS, and that tolerance was based not upon accelerated RES clearance of LPS, but upon development of resistance of the RES to LPS, leading to diminished release of endogenous pyrogens by RES cells. The liver, which contains the largest portion of the RES (Kupffer cells), was shown to be the organ primarily responsible for the production of fever when endotoxin is administered intravenously. This concept was supported by studies in humans with the collaboration of Henry N. Wagner, Jr., from The Johns Hopkins School of Medicine. RES activity was measured in volunteers as they were made tolerant to LPS. Tolerance was shown to occur in humans independently of any detectable increases in the generalized phagocytic activity of the RES.[4]

Typhoid Fever and Tularemia

Subsequently, we explored the role of endotoxin in mediating the physiologic derangements of typhoid fever and tularemia in man. These studies were carried out in conjunction with efforts to develop effective vaccines for these illnesses. We induced high levels of tolerance to LPS in fully informed volunteers by daily IV inoculations of purified LPS for several weeks, and observed that typhoid and tularemic illness could now be induced as readily as in nontolerant volunteers, with no mitigation of the febrile or toxic symptoms, even though the preinduced tolerance to LPS remained discernible during illness. We could also produce tolerance to endotoxin in other volunteers after they had become ill with typhoid fever and tularemia without affecting the fever or clinical course. We concluded from these studies that circulating endotoxin can play no major role in mediating the sustained febrile and toxic manifestations of these illnesses in man.[5-17] (Another group of investigators, using extremely sensitive in vitro assays not available during our studies, recently confirmed the absence of circulating endotoxin in patients with typhoid fever.) We subsequently demonstrated by intradermal inoculations of LPS and serial microscopy of biopsied specimens that tolerance to LPS does not occur to its local inflammatory inciting action in man even in the presence of tolerance to circulating LPS.[11] We concluded that endotoxin contributes to the pathogenesis of typhoid fever and tularemia by its persistent and highly potent local inflammatory inciting actions at the sites of bacterial lodgment.

Tolerance Acquisition

At about the same time as the above studies, we defined two phases of tolerance acquisition—early and late. The early phase was transient (hours to days), extended to LPS from all GNB, and secondary to refractoriness of the RES to the action of LPS. The later phase was prolonged (weeks to months), specific for LPS from a given serotype, and based upon antibodies to LPS. Some of this evidence was obtained by studies conducted in splenectomized volunteers. Since the spleen comprises only a minor portion of the RES (~5%) but is the major producer of circulating antibodies, following IV injections of particulate or colloidal antigens, we tested these concepts using splenectomized humans and rabbits. Initial pyrogenic and toxic responses were not affected by splenectomy, whereas antibody production and late-phase tolerance were markedly impaired. Our concept of early- and late-phase endotoxin tolerance is now fully accepted and frequently quoted by most investigators in the field.[6–10]

Gram-Negative Bacterial Sepsis

Our later studies addressed the role of LPS in GNB sepsis, and tested the hypothesis that antibodies to common core epitopes of LPS which are present in the outer membrane of all GNB, could provide broad-spectrum protection against GNB septic shock. We were the first to demonstrate that LPS does not play a major role in experimental GNB shock, but does so after antibiotic therapy is initiated. We presented these findings to the Association of American Physicians in 1984.[18] Serial blood measurements of LPS during murine GNB sepsis showed dramatic increases in circulating levels of LPS, commencing one hour after injection of aminoglycoside antibiotics or chloramphenicol and peaking at three hours, thereafter remaining sustained until *death*. This increase was shown not to result simply from impaired clearance of LPS from the circulation and to correlate with mortality. Little or no endotoxemia was seen in nonantibiotic-treated animals with

GNB sepsis, even when terminal. The liberation of LPS by antibiotics was also shown to correlate with the ability of corticosteroids, which were ineffective in the absence of antibiotics, to significantly protect against lethality. Timing was critical; the sooner the corticosteroid was administered, the more effective the protection. A number of investigators have subsequently confirmed the above observations.[18-20]

Our major effort in the last decades of our studies was concerned with testing the concept that antibodies raised to common core epitopes of LPS could provide broad-spectrum protection against GNB sepsis. Since the prevalence of GNB sepsis has increased markedly during the latter portion of this century because of increases in invasive procedures and immunosuppressive drugs, enormous sums have been spent by the National Institutes of Health (NIH) and by private industry (many billions) to develop antibodies that might be effective in reducing mortality from GNB sepsis. We were among the first to report studies that cast serious doubt on previously published numerous studies supporting the hypothesis that antibodies to LPS core epitopes were protective. We showed that most of these "positive" studies had inadequate controls, and that when proper controls were used, protection could not be demonstrated.[21,22] A final manuscript from our laboratory is a critical review of this subject.[23] Two internationally recognized authorities in the field, Drs. Ernst Th. Rietschel, Director of the Institute of Biomedical Research, Borstel, Germany, and Robert S. Munford, Professor of Medicine at the University of Texas Southwestern Medical Center at Dallas, Texas have sent congratulatory letters about this review, and for my receipt of the highest award that the International Endotoxin Society can bestow—Honorary Lifetime Membership. I shall cherish these letters throughout my retirement years.

ACKNOWLEDGMENTS

I cannot close this sojourn without acknowledgments to those who helped so much with the work outlined above. I was extremely fortunate and privileged to have met Ted Woodward who gave me the opportunity to perform the above studies, and who encouraged and supported these efforts throughout our 30-plus years of professional association. He would often ask if there was anything else he could do to facilitate the research ac-

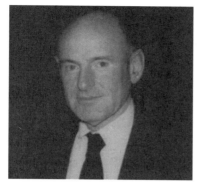

Sheldon E. Greisman, M.D.
Professor, Medicine, Physiology

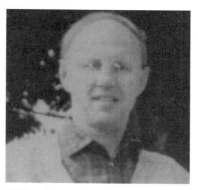

William E. Woodward, M.D.
Asst. prof. of Medicine,
Infectious Diseases

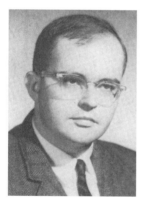

Frank A. Carozza, Jr., M.D.

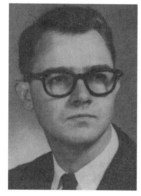

J. Bernard DuBuy, M.D.

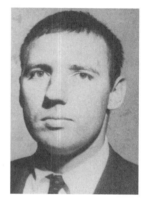

J. Dixon Hills, M.D.

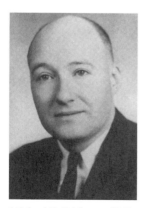

Michael B. Oldstone, M.D.

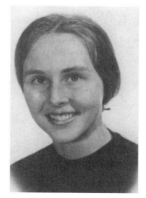

Celeste L. Woodward, M.D.

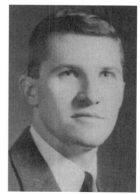

Edward J. Young, M.D.

tivities. He gave me complete freedom to pursue projects that undoubtedly seemed esoteric at the time and permitted me to also spend considerable amounts of time teaching in the Department of Physiology without asking anything in return. His philosophy, long since outmoded, was: Do what seems best for our medical school, not simply for our department. It is accurate to state that all the publications that came out of the Division of Infectious Diseases bearing my name are due to the encouragement and support of Ted Woodward. I would also like to acknowledge the encouragement and support of Charles L. Wisseman, Jr., and the assistance of two other key colleagues, Drs. Richard B. Hornick, Director of the Division of Infectious Diseases at the time, and Henry N. Wagner, Jr., at The Johns Hopkins School of Medicine, as well as the medical students who worked with me on these projects: Frank A. Carozza, Jr., J. Dixon Hills, Michael B. Oldstone, Celeste L. Woodward, William E. Woodward, J. Bernard Dubuy, Edward J. Young, and Curtis A. Johnston. These were truly golden years. Perhaps the most important accomplishment of all was the stimulation of these young students who today represent some of the finest physicians and scientists in our medical profession.

REFERENCES

1. Greisman SE. Capillary observations in patients with hemorrhagic fever and other infectious illnesses. J Clin Invest 1957;36:1688.

2. Greisman SE. On the collapse of bacterial endotoxin resistance following hemorrhage. J Exp Med 1960;112:257.

3. Greisman SE, Carozza FA Jr, Hills JD. Mechanisms of endotoxin tolerance. I. Relationship between tolerance and reticuloendothelial system phagocytic activity in the rabbit. J Exp Med 1963;117:663.

4. Greisman SE, Wagner HN Jr, Iio M, Hornick RB. Mechanisms of endotoxin tolerance. II. Relationship between endotoxin tolerance and reticuloendothelial system phagocytic activity in man. J Exp Med 1964;119:241.

5. Greisman SE, Woodward WE. Mechanisms of endotoxin tolerance. III. The refractory state during continuous intravenous infusions of endotoxin. J Exp Med 1965;121:911.

6. Greisman SE, Young EJ, Woodward WE. Mechanisms of endotoxin tolerance. IV. Specificity of the pyrogenic refractory state during continuous intravenous infusions of endotoxin. J Exp Med 1966;124:983.

7. Greisman SE, Young EJ, Carozza FA Jr. Mechanisms of endotoxin tolerance. V. Specificity of the early and late phases of pyrogenic tolerance. J Immunol 1969;103:1223.

8. Greisman SE, Woodward CL. Mechanisms of endotoxin tolerance. VII. The role of the liver. J Immunol 1970;105:1468.

9. Greisman SE, Young EJ, Dubuy JB. Mechanisms of endotoxin tolerance. VIII. Specificity of serum transfer. J Immunol 1973;111:1349.

10. Greisman SE, Young EJ, Workman JB, Ollodart MR, Hornick RB. Mechanisms of endotoxin tolerance: Role of the spleen. J Clin Invest 1975;56:1597.

11. Greisman SE, Hornick RB. Cellular inflammatory responses of man to bacterial endotoxins: a comparison with PPD and other bacterial antigens. J Immunol 1972;109:1210.

12. Greisman SE, Hornick RB. Mechanisms of endotoxin tolerance with special reference to man. J Infect Dis 1973;128 (Suppl.):265.

13. Johnston CA, Greisman SE. Mechanisms of endotoxin tolerance. In: Endotoxins: Pathophysiology of Endotoxin, Vol. II, Hinshaw, L.B., ed. Elsevier/North-Holland Biomedical Press, Amsterdam, 1983.

14. Greisman SE, Hornick RB, Carozza FA Jr, Woodward TE. The role of endotoxin during typhoid fever. I. Acquisition of tolerance to endotoxin. J Clin Invest 1963;42:1064.

15. Greisman SE, Hornick RB, Carozza FA Jr, Woodward TE. The role of endotoxin during typhoid fever. II. Alterations in cardiovascular responses to catecholamines. J Clin Invest 1964;43:986.

16. Greisman SE, Hornick RB, Carozza FA Jr, Woodward TE. The role of endotoxin during typhoid fever. III. Hyperreactivity to endotoxin during infection. J Clin Invest 1964;43:1747.

17. Greisman SE, Hornick RB, Wagner HN Jr, Woodward WE, Woodward TE. The role of endotoxin during typhoid fever and tularemia in man. IV. The integrity of the endotoxin tolerance mechanisms during infection. J Clin Invest 1969;48:613.

18. Johnston CA, Greisman SE. Endotoxemia induced by antibiotic therapy: a mechanism for adrenal corticosteroid protection in gram-negative sepsis. Trans Assoc Am Physicians 1984;97:172.

19. Greisman SE, Dubuy JB, Woodward CL. Experimental Gram-negative bacterial sepsis: Prevention of mortality not preventable by antibiotics alone. Infect Immun 1979;25:538.

20. Greisman SE. Experimental gram-negative bacterial sepsis: Optimal methylprednisolone requirements for prevention of mortality not preventable by antibiotics alone. Proc Soc Exp Biol Med 1982;170:436.

21. Greisman SE, DuBuy JB, Woodward CL. Experimental gram-negative bacterial sepsis: Reevaluation of the ability of rough mutant antisera to protect mice. Proc Soc Exp Biol Med 1978;158:482.

22. Greisman SE, Johnston CA. Failure of antisera to J5 and R595 rough mutants to reduce endotoxemic lethality. J Infect Dis 1988;157:54.

23. Greisman SE, Johnston CA. Evidence against the hypothesis that antibodies to the inner core of lipopolysaccharides in antisera raised by immunization with enterobacterial deep-rough mutants confer broad-spectrum protection during gram-negative bacterial sepsis. J Endotoxin Res 1997;4:133.

14

STUDIES OF PATHOGENESIS AND VACCINE CONTROL OF TYPHOID FEVER, TULAREMIA, SANDFLY FEVER, Q FEVER, BACILLARY DYSENTERY, CHOLERA, TOXIC DIARRHEA, RESPIRATORY VIRAL INFECTIONS, ROCKY MOUNTAIN SPOTTED FEVER, AND MALARIA

Richard B. Hornick, M.D., Chairman, 1963–1979

In 1959, after my two-year stint at Fort Detrick, Maryland, Dr. Woodward invited me to join the Department of Medicine instead of returning to the Osler Service of Johns Hopkins Hospital for a third year of residency. I was drafted from my residency to the Army as part of the Walter Reed Unit at Fort Detrick. Its mission was to develop vaccine and preventive measures against various infections thought to be potential bacteriologic warfare weapons; hence my decision to enter a career centered on infectious diseases. While at Fort Detrick, I worked with volunteers who participated in studies of induced tularemia conducted by Dr. Sam Saslaw at the University of Ohio, Ohio State

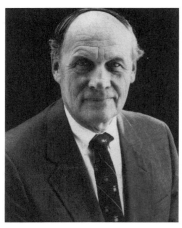

Richard B. Hornick, M.D.

Prison, Columbus, Ohio. The experience consisted of prison living for 24 hours, on and off.

Dr. Woodward served as a visiting consultant for the Walter Reed Unit, and he came to Fort Detrick on request. He saw one patient who was an employee with tularemic meningitis. Later, he attended a very ill patient with pulmonary anthrax—an electrician who, while changing fluorescent light bulbs, apparently inhaled spores from the laboratory.

My brief encounters with Dr. Woodward convinced me to accept the fellowship offered at Maryland, supported by the Armed Forces Epidemiological Board. The Board felt that more young physicians were needed for the growing field of infectious diseases, particularly those interested in the more exotic types of infection. I joined the division at the end of June 1959. Several weeks later, I was on a plane to Iran for the study of sandfly fever.

I accompanied Lt. Colonel Herbert Barnett from Walter Reed and his staff sergeant. We were housed in Tehran at the Pasteur Institute directed by Dr. Marcel Baltazard, a French investigator who was well known for his work on plague, and an old friend of Dr. Woodward. One of the many research projects at this institute was rabies. It was fascinating to observe the careful examination of numerous brains from dogs and wolves—animals that had bitten area residents.

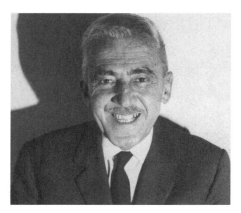

Marcel Baltazard, M.D.

Our group's objective was to obtain strains of sandfly fever viruses. I collected sand flies, attended various clinics in Tehran, and examined patients with early-onset febrile illness thought to be sandfly fever. Blood specimens were taken. Two strains of sandfly fever viruses came from these specimens. Visits to various villages were arranged. Permission from the village "chief" was sought for us to search for sand flies to develop a "clinic" to see patients. On July 4, after a meal with him, I developed dysentery caused by *Shigella sonnei*—an experience that prepared me for future volunteer studies. Sand flies were collected from the stables and houses. Blood was drawn from patients who visited our clinic. Many had chronic diseases that could not be altered by one visit and inadequate medical supplies. One marveled at the problems and tried to offer some solace.

Dr. Woodward and a group consisting of Joe Smadel, Ken Goodner, and John Dingle visited Tehran as a possible site for cholera research. They accompanied us on a field trip. In a village visited, a patient with cutaneous anthrax was encountered. Dr. Woodward's picture of that patient is a vivid reminder of diseases in Iran. I had authority to care for patients in a hospital ward about 10 kilometers south of Tehran. We borrowed an old Packard automobile from the Institute which allowed daily visits. Always there were 5 to 10 patients with typhoid fever who presented numerous complications. Also, there were many patients with various parasitic diseases. Some had superimposed protozoal diseases with typhoid. An unforgettable experience was to assist a young boy pass several roundworms from his mouth while acutely ill with typhoid fever. Apparently the worms were uncomfortable from the gastrointestinal inflammatory reaction and the chloramphenicol he received. He survived and recovered. I eventually took the boy to his home in the Packard. He had no idea where he lived; so it was an interesting problem to have him recognize the part of the city and street where he resided; his parents were not at home.

After three months in Iran, we went on a second field trip that involved Q fever, then regarded as a potential bacteriologic warfare threat. Dr. Fred McCrumb, an energetic and innovative investigator, was Director of the Infectious Diseases Division. Woodward and McCrumb arranged my trip to Montana in the winter of 1960 to determine the incidence of asymptomatic Q fever infection in sheep and cattle, and in the sheepherders and cowboys who worked with these animals. This research centered at the Rocky Mountain Laboratory in Hamilton, Montana. It involved laboratory work with Mike Gregg and other scientists using assays to detect Q fever antibody including milk specimens. Many human serum specimens showed antibodies to Q fever but no historical evidence of clinical illness. This experience introduced me to the rickettsial infections that played a significant role in later Baltimore studies.

On my return to Baltimore, plans had been completed to establish a clinical facility for ambulatory and inpatient studies using prison volunteers. New tularemia and typhoid vaccines were under intensive evaluation, particularly because of their military importance. While these negotiations were proceeding with the prison system, Dr. McCrumb and the team were evaluating attenuated measles strains. We vaccinated thousands of children primarily in St. Joseph, Missouri and in various sites throughout Maryland. I became adept at obtaining blood specimens from small children and became sensitized to their dislike of venapuncture.

These valuable field trials taught us the need for keeping accurate and follow-up data on participants. I returned to St. Joseph for 10 days to answer parents' questions about febrile reactions and other problems. This broadened my knowledge of pediatrics and human psychology. These measles vaccine field trials ultimately led to FDA approval and decline of incidence in the United States.

During this period, a more organized infectious disease clinical service was established, and consultative requests from various Baltimore hospitals provided excellent teaching material for students, residents, and fellows. Soon this highly successful program was enhanced even more by the recruitment of excellent physicians: Bert Dupont, Frank Calia, Mike Levine, Harold Standiford, and Steve Schimpff, to name a few. Dr. Woodward remained the ultimate clinical infectious disease expert to whom we turned for decisions on difficult diagnostic problems.

THE VOLUNTEER RESEARCH UNIT

With the help of Drs. Woodward and McCrumb, we met numerous times with officials of the Maryland prison system and various prisons in and around Baltimore and the surrounding counties. Drs. John King and Henry Thomas were very helpful in gaining approval for important decisions. We obtained permission to establish a small ward at the Maryland House of Correction at Jessup, Maryland. This initiated a long and very fruitful asso-

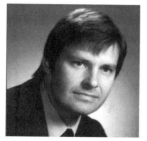
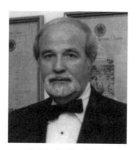
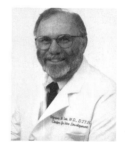

Herbert L. DuPont, M.D.   Frank M. Calia, M.D.   Myron M. Levine,
                          Prof. Medicine, Vice-   M.D., D.T.P.H.
                          Dean, School of Medicine

ciation with the Maryland penal system and resulted in the construction of a very modern ward and clinical facility. Funds were derived from contracts with the National Institutes of Health (NIH), World Health Organization (WHO), and the Department of Defense. Many studies reported in this discussion were conducted at those units. The unit was finally closed in 1974 (more on this later). For over a decade, we had the unique opportunity and privilege to conduct carefully designed studies of important infections in large groups of volunteers. This work delineated the quantitative effectiveness of vaccines and increased understanding of the pathogenesis of numerous infectious diseases.

Prior to the establishment of the specific ward, the prison hospital made four to six beds available in their annex for short-term studies. Earlier, prison volunteers were admitted to the University of Maryland Hospital for typhoid vaccine studies: a four-bed unit was used. This small unit permitted 1) very close control and continuous observation, 2) close scrutiny by various clinicians and nursing personnel, and 3) clear demonstration of a carefully conducted study.

TYPHOID FEVER AND VACCINE EFFICACY STUDIES

A primary objective was to determine the infectious dose of *Salmonella typhosa* required to induce typhoid fever in healthy adult volunteers and to determine if antibody levels had any effect on their subsequent clinical course. This information was needed to evaluate efficacy of available inactivated vaccines. The current data were unclear. Large-scale studies elsewhere reported some efficacy, but during World War II, there were many perceived vaccine failures. There was uncertainty regarding effectiveness, especially in persons living in nonendemic areas. We perceived that quantitative effectiveness of a vaccine could be obtained using a known infectious inocula in a small group of volunteers during a short period. Moreover, an effective antibiotic was available for ultimate control. The Quailes challenge strain used was obtained from a known typhoid carrier. It was cultured from bile taken during cholecystectomy performed to cure her carrier state (see earlier section). This strain was used subsequently in all volunteer studies. Other studies utilized the Ty2 standard strain and those lacking Vi antigen or "H" antigen.

The initial inoculum was selected to be 1×10^9. This dose had been used in a few volunteers by Dr. Woodward and his group several years previously using the Ty2 strain. Illness did not occur. Soon we found that the humanized Quailes strain at this dose caused illness in almost 100% of healthy volunteers. At the 10^7 level, the attack rate was about 50%. The majority of volunteers were challenged with 100,000 (10^5) organisms which produced illness in 25%–30% of those exposed. Very few volunteers developed illness at the 1000 (10^3) dose level, and most were asymptomatic. The 100,000 organism challenge was selected for the vaccine trials since we assumed this might be the causative dose under natural conditions. A comparison of incubation periods was analyzed, comparing our volunteer experience with selected epidemics such as the one in Zermatt, Switzerland. The incubation periods of the several groups was 10–13 days suggesting ingestion of 100,000 organisms. There was an inverse relationship between the size of the challenge dose and the incubation period. No other reliable data had surfaced regarding the size of inocula in nature. Some epidemiologists had suggested lower dosage inocula were more likely in nature than indicated in our dose response data.

The importance of the Vi antigen (Vi for virulence) causing illness was shown utilizing typhoid strains devoid of Vi antigen or lacking both the "H" (flagella antigen) and Vi antigens. Also the Zermatt strain (Vi containing) was tested. The challenge dose of each was 10^7 organisms. The Vi-containing strains caused illness in 51% of 47 volunteers, identical to the results obtained with the Quailes strain, while the non-Vi strains caused illness in 26% of 39 volunteers—a significant difference, p < .05.

Roger Miller, a fellow, studied Vi antigen virulence factors and discovered the inability of the phagocyte to consume oxygen after Quailes strain is ingested by leukocytes. Subsequently other investigators discovered that Vi antigens blocked C_3 fixation by *Salmonella typhi*. This action retards phagocytosis and slows the O_2 burst as expected with non-Vi strains.

Initially, three typhoid vaccines were evaluated: L, the phenol-treated classic vaccine that contains little Vi antigen; K, the acetone-treated vaccine that preserved more of the Vi antigen; and a purified Vi antigen. Each was administered to large numbers of volunteers. Subsequent challenge with 10^5 virulent organisms demonstrated good protection for those given K and L vaccines compared to controls. The Vi vaccine was not effective. The largest size inoculum, 10^9, overcame the induced immunity. In the later stages of these studies, the attack rate in controls increased from 25% to 30% with the 100,000 organism inoculum. Dr. William Woodward analyzed several hundred records and found a reasonable explanation: the initial group of volunteers were more likely to have served in the military (and received typhoid vaccine) and were born in areas when *S. typhi* and other *Salmonella* strains were more common than in subsequent decades. Hence, they had a higher level of acquired immunity. Volunteers in later stages of studies were, as a group, more susceptible because of less exposure to *Salmonella* antigens.

There was no correlation of Vi titers or O and H antibodies with subsequent clinical courses following challenge. The inverse relationship between the height of the titers prior to challenge and subsequent clinical course could not be established. There was no evidence that a larger inoculum produced a more severe case of typhoid fever.

A uniform illness occurred with large or small inocula. Blood cultures were performed at the end of expected incubation periods. Some asymptomatic volunteers were bacteremic; presumably they had excellent cellular immune mechanisms that prevented apparent illness.

Interest in pathogenesis of typhoid was the prime reason why volunteers gargled the infectious solution before swallowing. Early concepts suggested the pharynx as the portal of entry because of the tonsils and presence of pharyngitis. A few were given inocula via nasogastric tube directly to the stomach. Pharyngitis and pharyngeal lymph node enlargement developed early in the typhoid, whether the organisms were placed in the stomach or gargled and swallowed. The pharynx was not regarded as a portal of entry. Biopsy specimens of the duodenum obtained by Dr. Gene Gangarosa during the incubation period, showed increased inflammatory responses, which suggested penetration of S. *typhi* throughout the GI tract. No ulcerations or necrotic lesions were noted.

Initially, milk was used as the vector for S. *typhi* infection because it is a good buffer and permits the typhoid bacilli to transit the stomach. Attempts were made to recover S. *typhi* from the stomach juice following challenge. Viable organisms were isolated after 30 minutes and illness occurred in predicted numbers depending on the ingested dose (the concern regarding the gastric acid barrier and its effect on enteric pathogens was evaluated further in studies of *Shigella* and *Vibrio cholera* pathogens). In order to ensure reproducible challenges, the same protocol was followed in all studies. Under circumstances of challenge routines, reproducible results were obtained that permitted comparisons of the efficacy of typhoid vaccines. The data clarified vaccine efficacy and helped explain why induced immunity may be overcome by large inocula occurring in particular endemic areas.

These studies permitted assessment of immunity induced by typhoid fever, per se. Groups of volunteers previously ill or who failed to develop typhoid after challenge were rechallenged with an inoculum comparable to the first exposure. The attack rate was the same in the group with previous illness or resistant following the first challenge. Surprisingly, 25%–30% of volunteers experienced typhoid fever, as if they had never been exposed previously. Reasons are unclear but certainly may relate to defense mechanisms in the gastrointestinal tract where bacilli normally invade. Possibly the chloramphenicol impeded the development of complete immunity. Antibody titers were lower in the chloramphenicol group than in those treated with ampicillin.

Resistance factors in the intestine following exposure to virulent S. *typhi* are unclear. Not all exposed volunteers developed illness. Typhoid carriers shed voluminous numbers of pathogenic S. *typhosa* and remained well. This was the major stimulus, i.e., to stimulate the nonspecific and specific local immune GI tract mechanisms and prevent S. *typhi* from penetrating the epithelial border. Our volunteer model permitted testing of various oral vaccines. Killed oral vaccine showed no effect. A streptomycin-dependent attenuated vaccine was effective, but lost most of its efficacy when lyophilized. The Swiss Serum Institute developed a galactose-deficient attenuated living strain. We were able to administer the organism orally by slurry, and subsequently give a virulent challenge. These volunteers showed fewer positive stool cultures than others given the standard killed vaccines. Also, their degree of protection greatly exceeded that engendered by the killed vaccines. Later, Dr. Mike Levine conceived the necessity to encapsulate these organisms for ingestion by children. In Chile, there were good and some adverse results, because of difficulty in digestion of the capsules and their failure to release the attenuated living typhoid strain. This defect was corrected. The current attenuated encapsulated vaccine strain is now widely and safely used. Obviously, it does not provide absolute protection. This vaccine is now marketed in the United States as Vivotif.

Summary

The typhoid vaccine studies conducted over 13 years concluded with the development of an effective oral vaccine, due to the dedicated work of physicians, nurses, technicians, and volunteers. Complications in volunteers were minor; only one man developed acute cholecystitis, which was treated appropriately. There was no cross-contamination of any prison inmates or male nurses who worked for us. Emphasis on handwashing prevented any acquired infection. There was one laboratory-acquired infection. These studies required Saturday and Sunday coverage, and I occasionally took one or more of my children with me to the House of Correction in Jessup. On one such excursion, my daughter Marcie accompanied me into the laboratory where specimens were processed. Somehow, she placed her hand on a contaminated area and transferred organisms to her mouth. In about two weeks, she developed fever and was hospitalized by our pediatrician at the Union Memorial Hospital. He felt that she had an evolving leukemia or lymphoma, a frightening concept for her parents. I examined her closely and found two rose spots. Specimens yielded presumed *S. typhi* which did not agglutinate. After heating the bacteria, the Vi antigen disappeared and agglutination occurred. Her response to chloramphenicol was dramatic. Marcie subsequently volunteered for the cholera study 10 years later. She failed to acquire the disease.

During these studies, Dr. Merrill Snyder was a common denominator, who prepared each challenge inoculum. During the first five years of study, we checked the control inoculum for authentication of the number of *S. typhi* present. My travels to and from the prison involved transfer of unpleasant specimens for culture. Happily, recruited fellows were interested in these clinical studies

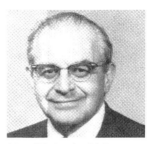

Merrill J. Snyder, Ph.D.
Prof. Medicine, Microbiology

and willingly participated in the care of inmates and administrative support. Care of volunteers on our wards was admirably performed by our own male nurses. Mr. Paul Sharpley was the first of many. Most were Army veterans and graduates from nursing schools. They were very helpful and took pride in their work. We were fortunate to have this excellent nursing support.

TULAREMIA

There was an obvious need to evaluate the living tularemic vaccine initially developed in Russia. These studies were among the first to be conducted at the House of Correction. Because of intense interest in biologic defense, these volunteer studies provided long-standing, effective association with investigators in the Fort Detrick Medical Unit and the Chemical Corps Division (Microbiology). Dr. Henry Eigelsbach characterized the various strains contained in the Russian living vaccine, and determined that only one was the critical antigen. Mr. William Griffith prepared the aerosols used in all studies designed to evaluate the respiratory route for vaccine administration. Several strains of *Francisella tularensis* were used: the virulent SCHU strain; an intermediate virulent strain, 425; and the avirulent LVS (live vaccine strain). Aerosol immunization and aerosol challenge studies were evaluated as well as intradermal infection. Small-particle aerosols were generated in the elaborate unit contained in a large eight-wheel trailer. Saslaw had shown that as few as 10–50 organisms, 3–5 micron size, caused tularemia using the aerosolized SCHU strain. Similar numbers caused infection when given subcutaneously. We evaluated the quantitative efficacy of the LVS-induced immunity relative to challenge with large doses of SCHU strain bacteria (e.g., 2500–3000 organisms). LVS induced full immunity against these and higher doses of this virulent strain. LVS and strain 425 were administered by aerosol in large doses. Inhaled in large doses of 10^6–10^8, it produced excellent immunity against a large SCHU challenge. However, the 10^8 dose of LVS caused a flu-like illness; three of 42 volunteers required streptomycin therapy. At the 10^6 level, reactions were milder without any disability. The aerosol route stimulated the best protection, but obviously the antigen was unsuitable for persons with chronic lung disease. No practical method for immunizing large groups, such as military personnel, was ever developed.

Strain 425 produced a mild form of tularemia which lasted four to seven days and did not require antibiotic therapy when 200–12,000 organisms were inhaled. Although strain 425 was not considered to be a suitable vaccine strain, it did stimulate excellent immunity against large SCHU aerosol challenges. Volunteers given large doses of LVS by aerosol were resistant to larger challenge doses of 425. This proved that LVS protected against the highly virulent SCHU strain (the North American strain) and the less virulent 425 strain, more like the Eurasian strains. LVS and the SCHU strain were given by mouth. One hundred million SCHU strain organisms produced illness when given orally. Half of the volunteers gargled and swallowed; others were given a gelatin capsule containing the organisms. Those who gargled developed large cervical lymph nodes which regressed rapidly with streptomycin therapy. The inoculum in capsules produced no reaction. All patients had an antibody response. The LVS strain showed similar but less severe illness; some patients required antibiotic treatment. Recipients of the oral LVS were immune following challenge if they developed antibodies with vaccination. These studies showed the feasibility of utilizing an unlikely portal of entry (oral) to safely immunize volunteers. Because of virulence of the SCHU strain and incidence of laboratory-acquired illness, we evaluated the possibility of human-to-human transmission. Liquid culture media was gargled by volunteers exposed in the trailer who expectorated into suitable containers. Sputum specimens were obtained. Cultures did not yield viable bacteria nor did inocula with sputum specimens cause illness in volunteers. How these pathogenic bacteria lost their virulence is unknown. Apparently, under natural conditions, patient-to-patient transfer does not occur.

SANDFLY FEVER

On my trip to Iran, strains of sandfly fever were isolated from various fly collections. Blood specimens collected from clinic patients often were positive for two strains of sandfly viruses. These strains were subsequently used to challenge volunteers as part of a vaccine trial. Volunteers developed a classic three-day febrile illness, self-limiting but minimally debilitating, like influenza. During these fever virus studies, Dr. Henry Wagner of the Johns Hopkins Department of Radiology (a former collaborator) studied the clearance of radio-tagged albumen from the reticuloendothelial (RES) system. This procedure helped quantitate RES system function. During the acute phases of tularemia and typhoid fever in volunteers, he had demonstrated an increase in RES activity. In sandfly fever virus infections, there was a marked inhibition of RES activity. This provided additional information about the inhibitory effects of viral agents on phagocytic cells. Subsequently, in rhinovirus infections, we found further evidence of inhibitory effects of viruses on ciliary epithelial cells. Dr. Wagner's group evaluated the clearance of a radio-tagged particle placed intranasally. During the incubation period of a common cold, he found that particles moved anteriorly rather than posteriorly. Obviously, the normal ciliary cell activity that clears the mucous membrane of the nose was blocked.

Q FEVER

Induced aerosol infections using *Coxiella burnetii* (Q fever) served to evaluate the efficacy of available Q fever vaccines. Initially, volunteers were exposed to a static aerosol at Fort Detrick. Permission was obtained to transport a busload of prison inmates to Frederick, Maryland for aerosol challenge in the Eight Ball. This million-cubic-foot aerosol chamber used a static aerosol different from the dynamic aerosol used in the trailer. I accompanied the inmates and remained with them while challenged in the Eight Ball chamber. They returned to the House of Correction for clinical and laboratory follow-up. The incubation period for Q fever was about 12 or 13 days; at the onset of fever, antibiotic treatment was promptly administered. Two challenges

in the Eight Ball were conducted. These studies showed the superior immunity induced by Phase I vaccine compared to Phase II, 0/13 ill versus 3/8, respectively, with 5/6 controls becoming ill. The 30-mg dose of Phase I vaccine was associated with reactions in 42% of 180 volunteers; 81% of 147 without baseline titers developed significant antibody increases at eight weeks. A similar challenge dose included 3500 GPIPID$_{50}$ as a dynamic aerosol. Phase I vaccine was a better preventive than Phase II; 2/19 versus 2/5, respectively, with 9/11 controls developing fever. The incubation period of 6.9 days was shorter in these controls compared to 12.2 days following the static challenge of 3000 GPIPID$_{50}$ dose. Reasons for this difference are unknown. In studies conducted in Montana, the question was frequently raised as to whether Q fever could be acquired by drinking milk contaminated with *C. burnetii*. Seven volunteers were fed 3500–350,000 GPIPID$_{50}$ doses without any evidence of infection. By contrast, the respiratory tract is obviously very susceptible to infection. Conceivably, these bacteria could be aerosolized when contaminated milk is poured into containers; viable organisms may then be inhaled.

ENTERIC PATHOGENS

Later studies permitted opportunities for evaluation of enteric pathogens. Dr. Sam Formal of the Walter Reed Institute of Research clarified pathogenesis of shigellosis in various animal species in an attempt to develop a vaccine. The opportunity was ripe for studies with shigella in volunteers. Dr. Bert DuPont was assigned to us by the Public Health Service which he served as Epidemiologic Intelligence Survey (EIS) officer at the Centers for Disease Control and Prevention (CDC). His major interest was enteric infections. During his tenure at Maryland, Bert contributed much to the understanding of pathogenesis of various enteric infections such as shigella, and several types of *Escherichia coli* (e.g., the entertoxigenic strains and penetrating types). Bert became actively involved in the shigella program, including the development of the vaccine. Attenuated vaccines did have some protective effect, but none seemed practical, and they did not achieve commercial status. Newer antibiotics were effective in preventing complications of dysentery. Small numbers of virulent shigella were shown to induce disease, and they were rel-

atively resistant to gastric acid. Bicarbonate was found to serve
as a buffer for the inoculum (see comments by Levine in Chapter
18). No reliable vaccine accrued from these studies, but much
was learned about virulence of the shigella species. Significant
leads followed regarding the induction of immunity against such
strains. Dr. DuPont worked in collaboration with Dr. Formal and
after completing his Public Health Service assignment, he joined
our medical facility.

Dr. Mike Levine, an EIS officer, joined our group and served
as an added stimulating investigator. He became involved actively in the studies on shigella and other enteric infections and in
the typhoid and cholera vaccine trials. Mike's strong interests in
tropical medicine greatly enhanced our international perspectives
and posture (see Chapter 18).

Problems regarding diarrheal disease in military forces in
Vietnam and elsewhere were instrumental in expansion of our related investigations. New information showed that toxins induced watery diarrhea. We evaluated various *E. coli* strains that
produced heat-labile and heat-stable toxins and the invasive
strains. They were shown to directly cause diarrhea, and the
clinical manifestations were clarified. A renewed interest in developing a cholera vaccine came in the late 1960s because of a widespread Southeast Asia pandemic. Effective vaccines were essential. Epidemiologic information revealed that U.S. citizens
residing in these endemic areas did not readily develop cholera.
This suggested that such personnel were less likely to ingest
V. cholerae compared to the indigenous population. Nevertheless, it seemed rational to evaluate the killed vaccines and obtain
better data of those immune mechanisms needed to resist infection with *V. cholerae* (full details are presented in other chapters).
In brief, large doses of Inaba and Ogawa strains are necessary to
cause clinical illness. Demonstration of the persistence of a gastric buffering effect induced by sodium bicarbonate in certain
volunteers increased the attack rate. Those volunteers able to se-
crete large volumes of gastric acid are more resistant to infection.
Dr. David Nalin showed that marijuana users were susceptible
because of its buffering effect.

The killed cholera vaccine showed little or no efficacy in preventing cholera in Americans who had no naturally acquired
background immunity. Cholera itself induced immunity against

species-specific re-challenges, but only partial protection against other strains of cholera or of *E. coli* heat-labile toxin-producing strains. Antitoxic immunity was not as effective as antibacterial immunity.

During the volunteer studies of enteric pathogens, various unique observations were conducted. Dr. Greisman showed that the cellular histologic reaction in volunteers following intradermal injections of endotoxin and purified protein derivative (PPD) differed. Endotoxin stimulated acute-phase reaction cells (polymorphonuclear cells) while the PPD recruited mononuclear cells. We realized that patients with typhoid fever who experienced intestinal perforation as a complication frequently had a monocytic cellular inflammatory response at the site of perforation. We became increasingly interested in the cellular components of diarrheal stools from patients infected with various enteric pathogens. John Harris, a summer student trainee, was assigned the responsibility of collecting specimens from volunteers and hospital patients with naturally acquired enteric infections. He examined the sediment of stool specimens to determine the cellular composition and added methylene blue stain to enable better detection. This is now a routine procedure in standard texts.

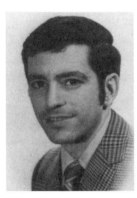
John Charles Harris

He reported a polymorphonuclear cell response from patients infected with strains that penetrated the epithelial lining of the intestinal tract (i.e., those likely to cause dysentery or systemic disease). These organisms are associated with sheets of white cells in the stool specimen. Other observations suggested that these cells were derived from the midcolon distally because of the short life span of white cells in the gut lumen. The finding of sheets of white cells in stools of patients with diarrhea is a differential finding between invasive pathogens and the usual toxigenic type. The latter do not cause an inflammatory response.

Dr. Robert Chanock and others of the NIH collaborated with us in helping develop vaccines for respiratory and gastrointestinal viral diseases. Collectively, we performed volunteer studies of rhino and influenza infections. An effective rhinovirus vaccine was developed that helped reduce respiratory tract infections in military recruits. An influenza vaccine that was administered as nose drops did not succeed. Now 25 years later, this route remains under investigation and shows promise.

Viral gastroenteritis was evaluated with NIH colleagues. Dr. Ray Dolin, an associate of Dr. Chanock and leader in this field, ultimately became Chairman of the Department of Medicine at the University of Rochester. With him, we evaluated the Norwalk agent; infected volunteers developed malabsorption abnormalities to certain lipids, particularly during their recovery phase. This was a new observation. Viruses similar to the Norwalk agent were identified that caused diarrheal outbreaks in young people.

RESPIRATORY TRACT INFECTIONS

The support of Dr. Yash Togo, our in-house virologist, enabled us to conduct influenza vaccine and chemotherapeutic trials. To induce influenza, careful screening of the volunteers for circulating antibodies was essential. Development of a reliable model made it possible to evaluate the therapeutic and prophylactic effects of amantadine. The preventive effect was excellent; little therapeutic action was demonstrated. Outbreaks of influenza at Jessup's House of Correction (see Chapter 15) and the Huntsville Prison in Texas permitted additional therapeutic trials.

Our experience with rhinoviruses permitted a prophylactic, double-blind study using Vitamin C. Stimulated by the wide press announcements reported by the Nobel Prize winner Linus Pauling, vitamin C was said to cure many illnesses such as cancer and the common cold. Funding was obtained. Three grams of vitamin C were given to one-half of infected volunteers starting two weeks prior to challenge and one week after challenge. Blind controls were used. Plasma, urine levels of vitamin C, and the amount of vitamin C in white cells were measured. Those who received vitamin C excreted large amounts in the urine. No differences were noted in virus excretion, antibody levels, or movement of the mucus blanket; Dr. Wagner and his team performed the latter studies. Subjective symptoms did not differ between the infected and control groups. While visiting in Baltimore, Dr. Pauling claimed that our challenge dose was too large, and therefore the study was not valid.

ROCKY MOUNTAIN SPOTTED FEVER

We evaluated Rocky Mountain spotted fever (RMSF) vaccines simply because of lack of evidence of effectiveness of available products and a perceived need for improvement. Dr. Charlie Wisseman, Irene Fabricant, and their group prepared the infectious inoculum for use in volunteers. The inoculum was injected subcutaneously to simulate a tick bite. A small number of rickettsiae induced infection, estimated to be 10 infectious organisms. Older vaccines that had been used for years were shown to prolong the incubation period and prevent relapses, but they did not prevent development of the illness. It was shown that RMSF responded rapidly to chloramphenicol given by mouth or intravenously. Recovered patients were shown to be solidly immune to re-infection.

MALARIA STUDIES CONDUCTED AT
THE MARYLAND HOUSE OF CORRECTION

The well-established volunteer study unit provided an opportunity to evaluate the chemotherapy and prevention of malaria. Falciparum strains of malaria had become resistant to chloroquine, and new therapeutic agents were essential. Colonel Herbert Barnett joined the Division along with other entomologists and established a mosquito-rearing facility on the fifth floor of the Bressler Building.

Transmission studies were initiated to establish an infectious model for vivax and falciparum malaria and thus enable evaluation of prophylaxis and therapy. Dr. Barnett transferred to Lahore, Pakistan to direct the tropical disease unit there: Dr. David Clyde, a recognized authority on malaria, was recruited to direct the malaria studies. Members of the Division of Infectious Diseases manned the clinical facility for the malaria trials, and cared for and treated the volunteers (see Chapter 16 for details of the work).

FINAL THOUGHTS

In retrospect it was stimulating and exciting to associate with fellows, residents, and faculty members along with colleagues at WRAIR, Fort Detrick, NIH, and my alma mater, Johns Hopkins. This was team work with exchange of ideas and technical material, all working collectively for the common goal of developing new prevention vaccines, better therapy, and fuller understanding of the mechanisms of infectious diseases. How refreshing it was to work with my dear friend, Dr. Shelly Greisman.

While stationed at Fort Derrick, senior investigators advised: "Don't waste your time working with endotoxin, it's so complex that no one is going to be able to figure it out." It was a pleasure to observe Greisman's clarification of this mystery substance and develop better understanding of its role in Gram-negative bacterial infections (see Chapter 13). Occasionally, we encountered difficulty with budgetary support, but Dr. Woodward always graciously helped to provide the means when needed, including contract input from the Department of Defense and pharmaceutical and other sources.

In the early 1970s, The American Civil Liberties Union (ACLU) caused a crisis, first through a long series of questions regarding the prison volunteer program. We provided complete details and answered every question raised. Subsequently, in 1974 the ACLU filed a malpractice suit against us. This soon became a class action suit involving inmates who had participated in our studies. This suit was based on the information provided in our response to their questions. We were then legally required to terminate the volunteer work using prisoners.

The ACLU actually enticed less than a dozen prison inmates to initiate the class action litigation. Included in the suit were the Governor of Maryland, President and Dean of Medical School of the University of Maryland, high officers of the Department of Defense, National Institutes of Health, and our staff members. Because of legal immunity, it was narrowed down to four defendants: Dr. Woodward, Director of the Program; Richard Hornick, as Responsible Investigator for contracts; and Bob Gillman and Bill Woodward, who were actively involved in the studies. Each was sued for a sum of approximately 75 million dollars.

After numerous depositions with lawyers, the suit came to a full-week trial before a federal judge in 1978. I testified for two full days and answered detailed questions from our lawyers from the State of Maryland Attorney General's Office. After testifying, I sat in the courtroom with our lawyers when Judge Kaufman announced, "Dr. Hornick, you have an emergency call, take it in my study." The call was from a Secret Service agent for whom we performed annual medical examinations. The emergency was his fear of impotence. While on the phone, I fiddled with the leg of the table and noted a loose bolt. It resembled a carriage bolt, so I pushed it in and reached around to tighten the nut while talking. Who would have guessed that it was a hidden alarm! A loud alarm resulted and immediately police and security rushed into the study with revolvers drawn; one had an automatic Winchester rifle. I sheepishly informed them of my mistake and after finishing the telephone conversation walked quietly into the courtroom with everyone in hilarious laughter. The judge had informed them that I had tripped the alarm. This made the day for everyone and helped lighten a tense atmosphere. Bob Gilman, under cross-examination, very vividly described how inmate volunteers were well informed of all details and possible complications. Bill Woodward carefully described the medical care, special technical and laboratory procedures used, and important follow-up information. Ted Woodward, the last to testify, was cross-examined by ACLU lawyers, and his attorney, Mr. Gordon Power, and Judge Ralph Kaufman questioned him. As a World War I (WWI) veteran, the judge inquired about the value of vaccine used in WW I. When informed that "Judge, those available vaccines were of little more value than water," he chuckled.

Judge Kaufman concluded the case by remarking about the high quality of the research in prison inmates, the high value of this investigation to the public as well as the military service, and the high ethical standards employed, which included evidence of full informed consent without coercion. About a month later, his written decision was transmitted which pleased and relieved us greatly. The ACLU had succeeded, however, in its mission, which was to completely stop prison research in the United States.

I close with great pride and knowledge of the value of these historic studies. They have been published in leading national and international periodicals. Members of our group have received rightfully deserved recognition, and I continue to reflect upon these memorable experiences.

EDITORIAL COMMENT

Leonard J. Morse, a New Englander, graduated from the University of Maryland School of Medicine in 1955, and then served with distinction as house officer, ID fellow, and chief medical resident. While with us, Leonard contributed importantly to the laboratory and clinical studies involving measles, typhoid fever, and tularemia vaccines. This experience was followed by his appointment to the Viral Diseases Section of WRAIR which provided him overseas research experience in Thailand and the

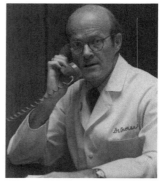

Leonard J. Morse, M.D.,
Former Chief Resident-Fellow

Philippines. While in the military service, Leonard helped perform pioneer studies of hemorrhagic fever and tick-borne encephalitis.

At Maryland, Leonard was a most affable colleague who insisted always in maintaining the highest clinical and ethical standards. He worked closely with Dick Hornick, Merrill Snyder, Yash Togo, and Ted Woodward, who all hold him in the highest regard.

Leonard returned to his native Worcester and fashioned a remarkable career which culminated in his academic appointment as full professor at the University of Worcester School of Medicine, chairman of several active hospital staffs, President of the Massachusetts Medical Society (1993), and member of the AMA Council on Ethical and Judicial Affairs (1996). His numerous publications on community health and practically applied preventive measures affirm, so well, his broad capacity as a physician and his scholarly traits.

PERTINENT REFERENCES BY FACULTY MEMBERS

Blacklow NR, Dolin R, Fedson DS, DuPont H, Northrup RS, Hornick RB, Chanock RM. Acute infectious nonbacterial gastroenteritis: Etiology and pathogenesis. Ann Intern Med 1972;76: 993–1008.

DuPont HL, Hornick RB, Dawkins AT, Heiner GG, Fabrikant IB, Wisseman CL Jr, Woodward TE. Rocky Mountain spotted fever: a comparative study of the active immunity induced by inactivated and viable pathogenic *Rickettsia rickettsii*. J Infect Dis 1973; 128(3):340–344.

DuPont HL, Hornick RB, Levin HS, Rapoport MI, Woodward TE. A study of Q fever hepatitis. Ann Intern Med 1971;74(2):198–206.

DuPont HL, Hornick RB, Snyder MJ, Dawkins AT, Heiner GG, Woodward TE. Studies of immunity in typhoid fever. Protection induced by killed oral antigens or primary infection. Bull WHO 1971;44(5): 667–672.

DuPont HL, Hornick RB, Snyder MJ, Formal SB. Study of Shigella vaccines in man. Symposia Series in Immunobiological Standardization. S. Karger AG: Basel, Switzerland, 1971;15:213–218.

DuPont HL, Hornick RB, Snyder MJ, Libonati JP, Formal SB, Gangarosa EJ. Immunity in Shigellosis. I. Response of man to attenuated strains of Shigella. J Infect Dis 1972;125(1):5–11.

DuPont HL, Hornick RB, Snyder MJ, Libonati JP, Woodward TE. Immunity in typhoid fever: Evaluation of live streptomycin-dependent vaccine. Antimicrob Agents Chemother 1970;10:236–239.

DuPont HL, Hornick RB, Weiss CF, Snyder MJ, Woodward TE. Evaluation of chloramphenicol acid succinate therapy for induced typhoid fever and Rocky Mountain spotted fever. N Engl J Med 1970; 282(2):53–57.

Gilman RH, Hornick RB, Woodward WE, DuPont HL, Snyder MJ, Levine MM, Libonati JP. Evaluation of a UDP-glucose-4-epimeraseless mutant of *Salmonella typhi* as a live oral vaccine. J Infect Dis 1977;136(6):717–723.

Harris JC, DuPont HL, Hornick RB. Fecal leukocytes in diarrheal illness. Ann Intern Med 1972;76(5):697–703.

Hornick RB, Dawkins AT, Eigelsbach HT, Tulis JJ. Oral tularemia vaccine in man. In: Antimicrobial Agents and Chemotherapy. Williams & Wilkins: Baltimore 1967, pp. 11–14.

Hornick RB, Eigelsbach HT. Aerogenic immunization of man with live tularemia vaccine. Bacteriol Rev 1966;30(3):532–538.

Hornick RB, Greisman SE, Woodward TE, DuPont HL, Dawkins AT, Snyder MJ. Typhoid fever: Pathogenesis and immunologic control. N Engl J Med 1970;283:686–691, 739–746.

Hornick RB, Music SI, Wenzel T, Cash R, Libonati JP, Snyder MJ, Woodward TE: The Broad Street pump revisited: Response of volunteers to ingested cholera vibrios. Bull NY Acad Med 1971; 47(10): 1181–1191.

Hornick RB, Schluederberg AE, McCrumb FR Jr. Vaccination with live attenuated measles virus. Am J Dis Child 1962;103:344–347.

Hornick RB, Togo Y, Mahler S, Iezzoni D. Evaluation of amantadine hydrochloride in the treatment of A₂ influenza disease. Bull WHO 1969;41:671–676.

Iio M, Wagner HN Jr, Hornick RB. Studies of reticuloendothelial system (RES). II. Changes in the function capacity of the RES in patients with certain infections. J Clin Invest 1963;42:427–434.

Kress S, Schluederberg AD, Hornick RB, Morse LJ, Cole J, Slater EA, McCrumb FR Jr. Studies with live, attenuated measles virus vaccine. II. Clinical and immunologic response of children in an open community. Am J Dis Child 1961;101:701–707.

Levine MM, DuPont HL, Hornick RB, Snyder MJ, Woodward TE, Gilman RH, Libonati JP. Attenuated streptomycin-dependent *Salmonella typhi* oral vaccine: Potential deleterious effects of lyophilization. J Infect Dis 1976;133(4):424–429.

Miller RM, Garbus J, Hornick RB. Lack of enhanced oxygen consumption by polymorphonuclear leukocytes on phagocytosis of virulent *Salmonella typhi*. Science 1972;175(25):1010–1011.

Snyder MJ, Hornick RB, McCrumb FR Jr, Morse LJ, Woodward TE. Asymptomatic typhoid bacteremia in volunteers. Antimicrob Agents Chemother 1963;604–607.

Perkins JC, Tucker DN, Knopf HL, Wenzel RP, Hornick RB, Kapikian AZ, Chanock RM. Evidence for protective effect of an inactivated rhinovirus vaccine administered by the nasal route. Am J Epidemiol 1969;90(4):319–326.

Togo Y, Hornick RB, Dawkins AT Jr. Studies on induced influenza in man. I. Double-blind studies designed to assess the prophylactic efficacy of amantadine hydrochloride against the A₂/Rockville/1/65 strain. 1968;203(13):1089–1094.

Togo Y, Hornick RB, Felitti VJ, Kaufman ML, Dawkins AT Jr, Klipe VE, Claghorn JL. Evaluation of therapeutic efficacy of amantadine in patients with naturally occurring A₂ influenza. JAMA 1970;211(7):1149–1156.

Eigelsbach HT, Hornick RB, Tulis JJ. Recent studies on live tularemia vaccine. Med Ann DC 1967;36(5):282–286.

15

STUDY OF HUMAN ANTIVIRAL VACCINES, CHEMOPROPHYLAXIS AND THERAPY FOR INFLUENZA, RHINOVIRUS INFECTIONS, AND DIAGNOSTIC VIROLOGY FOR MEASLES AND ENTEROVIRUSES

Yasushi Togo, M.D.

In 1955, while completing an invitation by the Japanese Medical Society to teach in various Japanese Medical Centers, Dr. Ted Woodward met my mentor, Dr. Shigeo Okinaka of the University of Tokyo Medical Center. This warm association led to my appointment in the Division of Infectious Diseases of the University of Maryland for specific training in virology. Drs. McCrumb, Parker, and Hornick were actively involved in clinical and laboratory investigative studies. Under their guidance, along with others, my 22 years at Maryland were not only satisfying, but shaped and developed my career. The privilege to work independently and freely under Dr. Hornick's guidance and assistance, along with many associates, provided affectionate memories never to be forgotten.

Equally cherished are my collaborative associations with Drs. Herbert L. Dupont, Lorraine Fiset, Joseph Libonati, Ann E.

Schluderberg, Merrill J. Snyder, and William E. Woodward. Dr. Suketami Tominaga and Mr. Philip K. Wilson of Dr. Klimpt's epidemiologic group assisted greatly in evaluating statistical data of vaccine trial studies. Many clinical fellows contributed importantly to our various vaccine and therapeutic test trials. Among those who excelled were Dr. Albert T. Dawkins, Jr. (Skip), Andrew R. Schwartz (Andy), and Elizabeth E. Kandell. Unlimited technical assistance was provided by Mrs. Margaret K. Ignatowski, Mrs. Helena P. Kulnich, and Mr. Yu Leung Lim.

The foundation of my testing was built from my review of pertinent bound publications given me by Dr. Hornick and my memory of the experiences as they evolved.

During my tenure with the Division of Infectious Diseases from 1956 to 1977, the projects in which I was privileged to participate actively were:

1. Efficacy evaluation of experimental antiviral agents in induced or naturally-occurring human influenza infections
2. Influenza vaccine studies
3. Efficacy evaluation of experimental antiviral agents in induced human rhinoviral infection
4. Rubeola and rubella hemagglutination-inhibition tests
5. Diagnostic virology

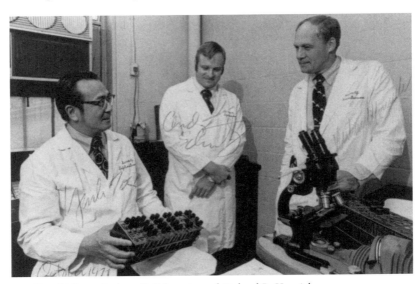

Drs. Yasushi Togo, Andrew R. Schwartz, and Richard B. Hornick

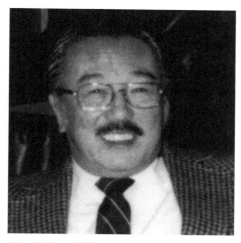

Yasushi Togo, M.D.
Assoc. Prof. Med. (Infectious Diseases)

EFFICACY EVALUATION OF EXPERIMENTAL
ANTIVIRAL AGENTS IN HUMAN INFLUENZA INFECTION

Acting on an invitation from the E.I. du Pont de Nemours & Co. in the mid-1960s, we conducted clinical trials in volunteers to assess the prophylactic efficacy of amantadine hydrochloride, a new anti-influenza drug. In previous trials with amantadine conducted by Dr. George G. Jackson of Illinois University and D.A.J. Tyrrell of the Common Cold Research Unit in England, attenuated type A influenza was the challenge virus. It was tested in volunteers who had pre-existing serum antibody against type A influenza. The data provided information limited to the extent of virus shedding and serum antibody responses. Drs. Dominic Iezzoni and Sarah Mahler, of the du Pont Laboratories, concurred with Dr. Hornick's and my suggestion to assess drug efficacy on clinical manifestations of induced influenza illness, as well as virus shedding and antibody responses. We required a fresh unattenuated strain of influenza virus isolate during recent outbreaks, and volunteers who lacked serum antibody for the challenge virus. To familiarize myself with the influenza virologic techniques, Dr. Mahler kindly arranged for me to work with Dr. J. T. Morris in the Division of Biological Standards at the National Institutes of Health (NIH). Here I learned the latest techniques and was given the A2/Rockville/1/65 strain. This served as the challenge strain and the antigen for serologic testing. It was maintained in human embryonic kidney cells.

The amantadine prophylactic double-blind, placebo-controlled trial conducted in 58 volunteers using the human influenza infectious model showed a clear-cut positive effect in all parameters. The data were well received at the IVth International Congress of Infectious Diseases (Munich) in April 1966, at ICAAC, and at other domestic and international meetings.

Encouraged by these results, Drs. Iezzoni and Mahler requested us to test rimantadine HC1 (an analogue of amantadine HCl) using the same test system. Our volunteer source at the Maryland House of Correction, susceptible to A2/Rockville/1/65 virus, was depleted. The rimantadine trial was conducted in 55 volunteers in Texas, and results were comparable to the amantadine study. The artificially induced influenza illness was severe in some cases, but was generally mild to moderate, and self-limited. All patients recovered without sequelae. These two clinical trials were published in JAMA.[1,2]. There were requests for over 2000 reprints. The editor provided me the lead plates used for preparing the tables and figures, which I had framed, with pride. Later in 1968, the therapeutic efficacy of amantadine in patient inmates with naturally-acquired A2 influenza was studied at Maryland and Texas prisons. Rapid defervescence and improvement in manifestations of illness occurred when patients were treated soon after the onset of illness. The causative viruses (A2/Maryland/1/68, A2/Texas/2/68) were equally isolated during the acute phase in both groups. Humoral as well as local (nasal secretions and sputum) antibody titers during the convalescence phase were comparable in the drug-treated and placebo groups.[3,4]

Because of the active interest of the pharmaceutical industry in developing new anti-influenza drugs and vaccines, we routinely isolated influenza A or B strains locally, and maintained samples of virus strains at $-70°C$. Newly isolated influenza strains were given to the WHO Collaborating Center for Influenza at the Center for Disease Control for WHO strain designation.

In 1970, Smith, Kline & French Laboratories requested us to evaluate their anti-influenzal agent, cyclooctylamine HCl (SK&F 23880A), administered by intranasal instillation to evaluate its prophylactic efficacy. A recent epidemic strain (A2/University of

Maryland/1/70) was used. This prophylactic topical treatment reduced the febrile course and virus excretion, but showed only minor effects on clinical signs in 16 volunteers. Serum and local antibody responses were significantly lower in the drug-treated group.[5]

In vitro studies with ribavirin (ICN 1229, virazole) showed inhibition of influenza A replication similar to amantadine HCl and cyclooctylamine HCl. Influenza B was also inhibited. In 29 volunteers who received ribavirin, amantadine HCl and placebo, amantadine showed the anticipated results, but ribavirin showed no effect. Likewise, ribavirin was not helpful in 18 volunteers challenged with A/Dunedin/73; similarly, there were only marginal effects against B/Georgia/26/74 challenge.[6]

During the period of testing in 1974 when the Jessup correctional facilities were unavailable, volunteer trials for influenza A were conducted in Florida and Arkansas under sponsorship of Lederle Laboratories. All laboratory specimens were transmitted to our unit for virus isolation and serologic testing.

As interest in development of anti-influenzal agents waned, ribavirin was the last anti-influenza chemoprophylactic or chemotherapeutic agent studied by us.[7,8]

During the early winter of 1970, I developed a severe flu-like illness which responded to Symmetrel (amantadine HCl); a nose swab sample yielded type A influenza (H3N2). Always when spraying aerosolized virus to volunteers, I wore a mask and goggles. How I remained susceptible in spite of constant exposure remains a mystery.

INFLUENZA VACCINE STUDIES

Smith, Kline & French Laboratories asked us to evaluate the immunogenic potency and safety of two live attenuated influenza vaccines developed in Belgium. These were recombinant vaccines containing live antigens from England, Hong Kong, and Russia. Several trials under our auspices were conducted during 1973–1974 at the Veterans Administration Center, Martinsburg, West Virginia and at the San Juan Veterans Administration facility in Puerto Rico.

Approximately 250 elderly persons, including some with cardiac, pulmonary, and metabolic disorders, were included. In each study, one half of the participants received one injection of killed parenteral vaccine, Alice vaccine (A/England/42/72 and B/Massachusetts/71). At Martinsburg, the remaining half received one dose of the Alice vaccine, and at San Juan, two doses were given at an interval of two weeks.[9,10] In a third study conducted at the Jessup correctional facility, 94 and 97 healthy men received the vaccine and placebo, respectively.[11] In all studies, the Alice vaccine was well tolerated with good local and systemic antibody responses. Subsequently, the Alice vaccine was licensed in Europe. The influenza B virus vaccine (R75) was given in two doses at two-week intervals and tested blindly in 43 seronegative adults.[12] There was no difference in the clinical indices, and 76% of vaccinees seroconverted.

The following three trial studies were conducted jointly with the National Institute of Allergy and Infectious Diseases (NIAID), of the NIH:

1. Respiratory secretory antibody (IgA class) responses were compared in volunteers who received live or killed influenza virus intranasally and those who were injected with killed virus. Intranasal administration of live or killed virus gave rise to higher antibody titers that lasted longer.[13–16]
2. A low-temperature (25°C)-adapted live influenza A2/AA/6/60 virus vaccine, cold-adapted virus by Dr. Hunein F. Massab, was evaluated in 13 volunteers with pre-existing antibodies. Significant serum and secretory antibody responses were noted.[17]
3. Live, oral, enteric-coated, monovalent vaccines containing types 1, 2, and 5 adenoviruses and a placebo were studied in 9, 8, 11, and 10 seronegative adult volunteers, respectively. These adenovirus types had been previously reported as the predominant isolates in pediatric respiratory tract infections caused by adenoviruses. Excretion of vaccine-type viruses were detected and, in over two-thirds of the vaccinees, a rise in serum neutralizing antibody titer against the respective vaccine virus was noted.[18]

EFFICACY EVALUATION OF EXPERIMENTAL ANTIVIRAL AGENTS IN INDUCED HUMAN RHINOVIRAL INFECTION

In the 1970s, the rhinovirus group included nearly 100 distinct serotypes, and no local or nationwide survey data regarding prevalent serotypes were available. Attempts to produce a multi-valent vaccine were out of the question. All investigators eagerly sought specific chemotherapy for the common cold, and how to eliminate causative agents such as rhinoviruses. Smith, Kline & French Laboratories and others developed candidate drugs that required evaluations in human testing.

We made a large pool containing a second passage rhinovirus 44 (from a throat washing supplied by Dr. A.Z. Kapikian, NIAID, NIH) in a rolling WI-38 diploid cell culture. Later, rhinovirus 24 and 32 challenge pools were similarly prepared. These challenge viruses, inoculated intranasally in volunteers, with minimal or no homologous serum-neutralizing antibodies, caused nasal congestion, rhinorrhea, sneezing, sore throat, mild cough, pharyngitis, and other respiratory signs within 24 hours. The infections peaked on the third to fourth post-challenge day before tapering off.

Various triazinoindole drugs were developed by Smith, Kline & French Laboratories for clinical evaluation. Drug administration of various suspensions of a micronized powder were instilled into the nostrils of volunteers two days before virus challenge and continued for five days. Controlled studies in Jessup prison volunteers showed no differences in the frequency and severity of clinical illness, virus shedding patterns, and serum and secretory antibody responses.[19]

The action of ascorbic acid (vitamin C) in prevention and cure of the common cold was very controversial. To assess its efficacy in induced rhinovirus infection, 11 men received a 1-gram tablet of ascorbic acid and 10 men received a placebo, three times daily for two weeks. Rhinovirus 44 was administered. Each volunteer continued the same vitamin dose for one week post-challenge. All men developed colds and no difference was noted regarding symptom scores, antibody responses, and virus shedding pattern between the two groups. In this study, the mucociliary flow rate was found to decrease during infection in both groups, but was not affected by ingestion of ascorbic acid. This study was conducted at the Jessup Correctional Institution and was supported by Hoffmann-La Roche, Inc.[20,21] Dr. Linus Pauling visited Baltimore when Dr. Hornick presented the data to him.

Prophylactic administration of 3,4-dihydro-1-isoquinoline-acetamide HCl (DIQA, Hoffmann-La Roche, Inc.) against rhinovirus 24 challenge was evaluated in two trials including 16 men and 5 prison volunteers. Ten men received a DIQA capsule (500 mg) and 11, received a placebo. Utilizing various doses given over five days, the DIQA therapy appeared to suppress the cold syndrome and reduce virus excretion, although its effect was marginal. The same marginal effects of isoprinosine and guanidine derivatives for prevention of rhinovirus infections were noted.[22-24]

RUBEOLA AND RUBELLA HEMAGGLUTINATION-INHIBITION TESTS

During clinical trials of a live, attenuated canine renal cell culture-derived measles (the Edmonton strain) vaccine in children, antibody responses of vaccine recipients were tested by the serum neutralization and complement-fixation tests.[25,26] The serum neutralization test was sensitive, reproducible, and reliable, but time-consuming, cumbersome, and expensive. In the early 1960s, a few papers dealing with the measles HI test indicated that the erythrocytes of African green monkeys were highly sensitive to measles hemagglutinin. We found that the HI test using erythrocytes of *Cercopithecus albiguaris* and the antigen prepared in H.Ep.#2 cell culture was a sensitive, reproducible, quick, and easy-to-run test with good correlation with the neutralization test.[27]

The Cendehill strain of rubella vaccine was made at R.I.T. (Recherche Industrie et Thérapeutique) In the mid-1960s, Smith, Kline & French Laboratories conducted a wide-scale potency and safety testing of the vaccine in children.[28] Prior to this, we tested this vaccine in a pediatric population at the Rosewood State Hospital, Owings Mills, Maryland and in adult women including seronegative student nurses and inmates at the Maryland House of Correction for Women, Jessup, Maryland.

Open-field trials at parochial schools in Baltimore City included 4000 children, and those at Army hospitals at Fort Mead and the Aberdeen Proving Ground included over 2700 children. All serum samples, mostly paired, were tested for HI antibody titers by microplate technique in our laboratory. Duplicate serum samples were tested at the Smith, Kline & French Laboratories. The results obtained in two laboratories were in complete agreement, and Smith, Kline & French later continued to send us many serum samples collected for HI tests in studies performed by other investigators.

DIAGNOSTIC VIROLOGY

In the late 1950s, Dr. McCrumb asked me to conduct a survey of viral aseptic meningitis. Poliomyelitis was very prevalent, and a large ward at Baltimore City Hospital was filled with patients in "iron lungs." Using newly developed tissue culture techniques, a variety of new viruses, especially these of enteric and respiratory types regarded of clinical importance, were appearing. We received clinical samples for virus isolation and paired serum specimens from hospitals throughout Baltimore. In the following decade, we identified about 100 cases of aseptic meningitis, encephalitis, and other infections caused by Coxsackie and ECHO viruses. The interesting informative cases were published.[29-36] In the late 1960s, the Maryland State Health Department started a summary evaluation of enterovirus infections in Maryland, to which report our case experience was contributed.

While engaged in volunteer studies on two occasions, I was visited by FDA inspectors as one of 100 investigators evaluated. They carefully evaluated our protocols, case reports, records, written informed consent forms signed by participants, correspondence with the University of Maryland Committee on Clinical Investigation and sponsors of the studies, responsible investigators, and other details. On each occasion, they were thorough and congratulated us for our carefully designed work and all pertinent records that were orderly filed.

EDITORIAL COMMENT

As shown by the following list of references, it is clear that Dr. Togo and the group made significant contributions to vaccinology, chemoprophylaxis, and chemotherapy of respiratory virus infections and to diagnostic procedures. Yash and his wife Kay were active participants in Division activities, and Kay was often "the hit of the evening" with her Japanese gown and obi.

We enjoyed close affiliation with Merck and Company during this period. They requested help in recruitment of a medical scientist well versed in infectious diseases who spoke Japanese. Yash was "the made-to-order person for the task" and when based in Tokyo during the next decade as Head of Research and Development for Merck, he established important linkages with academic centers. Pharmaceutical outlets were exploited, and marketing programs were greatly expanded, as was support of research. In 1990, the Togos returned to their Baltimore home for retirement and the enjoyment of their family and grandchildren.

REFERENCES

1. Togo Y, Hornick RB, Dawkins AT Jr. Studies on induced influenza in man. I. Double-blind studies designed to assess the prophylactic efficacy of amantadine hydrochloride against the A2/Rockville/1/65 strain. JAMA 1968;203:1089–1094.

2. Dawkins AT Jr, Gallager LR, Togo Y, Hornick RB, Harris BA. Studies on induced influenza in man. II. Double-blind study designed to assess the prophylactic efficacy of an analogue of amantadine hydrochloride (Rimantadine). JAMA 1968;203:1095–1099.

3. Togo Y, Hornick RB, Felitti VJ, Kaufman ML, Dawkins AT Jr, Kilpe VE, Claghorn JL. Evaluation of therapeutic efficacy of amantadine in patients with naturally occurring A2 influenza. JAMA 1970;211: 1149–1156.

4. Hornick RB, Togo Y, Mahler SA, Iezzoni D. Evaluation of amantadine hydrochloride in the treatment of A2 influenzal disease. Ann NY Acad Sci 1970;173:10–19.

5. Togo Y, Schwartz AR, Tominaga S, Hornick RB. Intranasal cyclooctylamine in the prevention of experimental human influenza. JAMA 1972;220:837–841.

6. Togo Y. In vitro effect of Virazole against influenza viruses. Antimicrob Agents Chemother 1973;4:641–642.

7. Togo Y, McCracken EA. Double-blind clinical assessment of ribavirin (Virazole) in the prevention of induced infection with type B influenza virus. J Infect Dis 1976;133 (Suppl):A109–A113.

8. Cohen A, Togo Y, Khakoo R, Waldman R, Sigel M. Comparative clinical and laboratory evaluation of the prophylactic capacity of ribavirin, amantadine hydrochloride, and placebo in induced human influenza type A. J Infect Dis 1976;133 (Suppl):A114–A120.

9. Miller LW, Hume EB, O'Brien FR, Togo Y, Hornick RB. Alice strain live attenuated influenza (H3N2) vaccine in an elderly population. Am J Epidemiol 1975;101:340–346.

10. Miller LW, Togo Y, Hornick RB. Clinical and serological effects of Alice strain live attenuated influenza A (H3N2) virus vaccine in an adult population. Med Microbiol Immun 1975;162:15–21.

11. Perez-Rodriguez F, Bermudez RH, Brau CJ, Togo Y. Attenuated influenza virus intranasal vaccine in a high risk male population. Bol Asso Med Puerto Rico 1975;67:376–380.

12. Miller LW, Togo Y, Hornick RB. Clinical and serological effects of live attenuated serum inhibitor-resistant influenza B vaccine in sero-negative adults. J Med Virol 1977;1:193–199.

13. Mann JJ, Waldman RH, Togo Y, Heiner GG, Dawkins AT Jr, Kasel JA. Antibody response in respiratory secretions of volunteers given live and dead influenza virus. J Immunol 1968;100:726–735.

14. Waldman RH, Kasel JA, Fulk RV, Togo Y, Hornick RB, Heiner GG, Dawkins AT Jr. Influenza antibody in human respiratory secretions after subcutaneous or respiratory immunization with inactivated virus. Nature 1968;218:594–595.

15. Kasel JA, Hume EB, Fulk RV, Togo Y, Huber M, Hornick RB. Antibody responses in nasal secretions and serum of elderly persons following local or parenteral administration of inactivated influenza virus vaccine. J Immunol 1969;102:555–562.

16. Rossen RD, Butler WT, Waldman RH, Alford RH, Hornick RB, Togo Y, Kasel JA. The proteins in nasal secretion. II. A longitudinal study of IgA and neutralizing antibody levels in nasal washings from men infected with influenza virus. JAMA 1970;211:1157–1161.

17. Kitayama T, Togo Y, Hornick RB, Friedwald WT. Low-temperature-adapted influenza A2/AA/6/60 virus vaccine in man. Infect Immun 1973;77:119–122.

18. Schwartz AR, Togo Y, Hornick RB. Clinical evaluation of live, oral types 1, 2 and 5 adenovirus vaccines. Am Rev Respir Dis 1974;109:223–238.

19. Togo Y, Schwartz AR, Hornick RB. Failure of a 3-substituted triazino-indole in the prevention of experimental human rhinovirus infection. Chemotherapy 1973;18:12–26.

20. Schwartz AR, Togo Y, Hornick RB, Tominaga S, Gleckman RA. Evaluation of the efficacy of ascorbic acid in prophylaxis of induced rhinovirus 44 infection in man. J Infect Dis 1973;128:500–505.

21. Sakakura Y, Sasaki Y, Hornick RB, Togo Y, Schwartz AR, Wagner HN Jr, Proctor DF. Mucocilliary function during experimentally induced rhinovirus infection in man. Ann Otol Rhinol Laryngol 1973;82:203–211.

22. Togo Y, Schwartz AR, Hornick RB. Antiviral effect of 3, 4-dihydro-1-isoquinolineacetamide hydrochloride in experimental

human rhinovirus infection. Antimicrob Agents and Chemother 1973; 4:612–616.

23. Pachuta DM, Togo Y, Hornick RB, Schwartz AR, Tominaga S. Evaluation of isoprinosine in experimental human rhinovirus infection. Antimicrob Agents Chemother 1974;5:403–408.

24. Togo Y, Durr FE, Laurenzana DA. Clinical evaluation of prophylactic intranasal 1-phenyl-3-(4-phenyl-2-triazolyl) guanidine (CL 88,277) medication against rhinovirus 44 challenge. Med Microbiol Immun 1977;163:37–44.

25. McCrumb FR Jr, Bulkeley JT, Hornick RB, Snyder MJ, Togo Y. Clinical trials with living, attenuated measles-virus vaccines. Am J Public Health 1962;52:11–15.

26. McCrumb FR Jr, Bulkeley JT, Hornick RB, Snyder MJ, Togo Y. Globulin-modified, live attenuated measles-virus vaccination. Am J Dis Child 1962;103:350–353.

27. Togo Y. Hemagglutination-inhibition test in the study of measles immunity. Am J Hyg 1964;79:250–259.

28. Kilpe VE, Sabundayo RM, Schwartz AR, Togo Y, Hornick RB. Clinical studies with the Cendehill strain of attenuated rubella vaccine. Antimicrob Agents Chemother 1969;352–356.

29. Woodward TE, McCrumb FR Jr, Carey TN, Togo Y. Viral and rickettsial causes of cardiac diseases, including the Coxsackie virus etiology and pericarditis and myocarditis. Ann Intern Med 1960;53: 1130–1150.

30. Robino G, Perlman A, Togo Y, Reback J. Fatal neonatal infection due to Coxsackie B2 virus. J Pediatr 1962;61:911–918.

31. Walker SH, Togo Y. Encephalitis due to group B, type 5 Coxsackie virus. Am J Dis Child 1963;105:209–212.

32. Walker SH, Togo Y, Keefer MM. Coxsackie virus group A, type 7 infection in Maryland. Maryland State Med J 1967;16:73074.

33. Woodward TE, Togo Y, Lee YC, Hornick RB. Specific microbial infections of the myocardium and pericardium. A study of 82 patients. Arch Intern Med 1967;120:270–279.

34. Music SI, Fine EM, Togo Y. Zoster-like disease in the newborn due to herpes simplex virus. N Engl J Med 1971;284:24–26.

35. Wald ER, Levine MM, Togo Y. Concomitant varicella and staphylococcal scalded skin syndrome. J Pediatr 1973;83:1017–1019.

36. Levine MM, Togo Y, Wald ER. Practicability of prospective influenza surveillance. Am J Epidemiol 1974;100:272–276.

16

MALARIA STUDIES AT THE UNIVERSITY OF MARYLAND, 1964–1975

David Clyde, M.D.

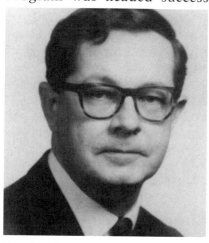

David F. Clyde, M.D., Ph.D.

Closely affiliated with the Division of Infectious Diseases in the old Bressler Building and at the medical research ward at Jessup, the onshore part of the International Health Program was headed successively by Drs. Fred McCrumb, Christopher Klimt, and David F. Clyde [the overseas part being the International Centers for Medical Research and Training (ICMRT) in Lahore, with a later offshoot in Bahia, Brazil under Herbert Barnett]. From inception of studies in the early 1960s, a principal part of the onshore work involved research into malaria, supported largely by contracts with Army R&D Command through Walter Reed Army Institute of Research (WRAIR).

This program had for its main thrust the testing in volunteers of candidate chemotherapeutic agents being developed at WRAIR and, as a sideline, the initial human trials of antimalarial immunogens. In support of the work, Dr. Richard Baker opened a mosquito insectary in the Bressler Building, breeding a variety of anophelines, notably important malaria vectors representative of different world regions: for North America, *Anopheles quadrimaculatus* and *A. freeborni*; Africa, *A. gambiae*; Pakistan and India, *A. stephensi*; Southeast Asia, *A. sundaicus* and (with difficulty) *A. balabacensis*; Europe, *A. maculipennis*; and Central and South America, *A. darlingi* and *A. albimanus*. It soon became apparent that problems in maintaining so varied a menagerie necessitated selection of *A. gambiae* and *A. stephensi* as easiest to maintain and use effectively in the malaria transmission studies.

Vincent (Vince) McCarthy worked closely with Dr. Richard Baker and made important observations at the mosquito insectary in Lahore (Pakistan Medical Research Center) and Baltimore (Bressler Building). The successful breeding of anopheline mosquitoes was essential for conducting drug testing and transmission studies. The relative degrees of infection, transmission of drug-resistant strains of plasmodia, and evaluation of immunity were dependent upon a reliable source of mosquito vectors.

Although maximum security measures were enforced to prevent escape of these mosquitoes at their home in the Bressler Building and in the facility at Jessup, where they were fed in small containers placed on the arms of volunteers, either to pick up the infective gametocyte stages of the malaria parasite in the blood meals or to transmit the sporozoite stages back to the volunteers, the mosquitoes had to be transported frequently between the two centers in cages, along the fast Baltimore-Washington Parkway. The possibility of an automobile accident en route, with escape of infected mosquitoes into the Maryland countryside, had to be borne in mind and, although remote, was sufficiently plausible that a decision was made by the licensing authority, the Centers for Disease Control, that the *A. gambiae* colony should be suppressed. (The ability of this most dangerous vector to establish itself in new regions was notorious, its classic migration from Africa to Brazil having been most costly, in terms of malaria morbidity and international efforts in the 1940s— eventually successful—to eradicate it from Brazil.) Accordingly, the transmission studies at Jessup proceeded using *A. stephensi*. When Baker was transferred to the ICMRT in Lahore to commence his lengthy series of studies into genetics of culicine mosquitoes, Dr. Vincent C. McCarthy, who had been studying ticks in Pakistan, came from Lahore to take over the Bressler insectory, which he ran until the closure of the program in the mid-1970s. Some studies of the transmission efficacy of the mosquitoes were published.[1–3]

CHEMOTHERAPEUTIC TRIALS

The principal work of the onshore malaria program consisted of trials of candidate antimalarial drugs provided by WRAIR. A number of collaborators at other institutions received samples from these studies for their individual research. The work was undertaken among adult volunteers at Jessup, malaria being transmitted by both the standardized methods: through mosquitos previously infected from gametocyte carriers of the species *Plasmodium falciparum* and *P. vivax*, and by blood from acutely infected volunteers (blood culture techniques for *P. falciparum* had not yet been developed). The work was included in the general infectious diseases program being undertaken at Jessup by Dr. Richard Hornick and his staff; the volunteers had to meet the same rigorous ethical requirements and health screening, and were attended by the same staff including nurses and a laboratory technician stationed at Jessup.

The importance of these chemotherapeutic trials was enhanced by the urgent need for a new generation of antimalarial drugs to replace chloroquine, to which *P. falciparum* was becoming resistant in Southeast Asia and South America with dire consequences for the management of this most serious form of the disease among military and civilians alike. Two of the candidate compounds, coded WR30090 and WR33063, were used in tests which proved to be the first prophylactic and therapeutic tests in humans leading to the provision and worldwide deployment of mefloquine and halofantrine.[4]

CLINICAL STUDIES OF DRUG-RESISTANT MALARIA

A part of the clinical studies at Jessup involved evaluation of the drug-resistant characteristics of strains of *P. falciparum* brought back from several countries of Southeast Asia. The problem, developing during the late 1950s on the border of Thailand and Cambodia (and soon after in Colombia and Venezuela) and involving progressive loss of parasite sensitivity to the universally used drug chloroquine, and sometimes to pyrimethamine and quinine, became increasingly serious as the resistant strains spread rapidly during the 1960s and 1970s throughout the region. It constituted a major impediment to concurrent military operations in Vietnam, as well as to success of the worldwide malaria eradication campaign being conducted by the World Health Organization. The strains were collected by Clyde from patients in the suspected foci, and brought back to Maryland in blood stored in tubes in a thermos flask packed with carbon dioxide ice. The journeys had to be routed through friendly institutes in Kuala Lumpur, Manila, and Honolulu where the dry ice could be replenished. Since that was a period of justified fear of aircraft hijacking and bomb threats, even the production of the necessary CDC import certificates for infective biologic materials did not always allay the suspicions of airport security personnel who (at a safe distance) made the carrier unstop the steaming flasks.

Safely brought to Baltimore, prior to inoculation into a single volunteer for propagation, the blood samples were tested for hepatitis virus. No adverse effects (other than the induced malaria) occurred in any of these men.[5]

CLINICAL STUDIES OF *VIVAX* MALARIA

Although considerably less important than *falciparum* malaria, infections caused by *P. vivax* were studied in the program. The incubation and relapse patterns of a strain from Vietnam were compared with those of the notorious New Guinea (Chesson) strain, and the anti-relapse efficacy of a 7-day course of primaquine at double dosage was found to be as effective as the standard course of 14 days. A study in collaboration with Dr. Louis Miller of the NIH conclusively proved that absence of erythrocyte membrane Duffy factor was the reason why Africans and their descendents in America did not contract *vivax* malaria. In this double-blinded study, the infections were induced (or failed to develop) in a number of African American and Caucasian volunteers at Jessup, while blood for Duffy genotyping was sent to the NIH.[6-8]

IMMUNIZATION AGAINST
MALARIA: THE FIRST SUCCESSFUL TRIALS

It had been shown since the late 1930s that live irradiated avian and rodent malarial sporozoites, if inoculated in very large numbers, could immunize the recipient against homologous species challenge by sporozoites (much research using killed parasites had been fruitless). Arising from work by Ruth and Victor Nussenzweig and J.P. Vanderberg at New York University in the late 1960s, in which whole sporozoite-bearing mosquitoes were irradiated and successfully immunized the rodents on which they fed, in 1970 Dr. Harry Most (an eminent physician and former health officer of New York City and consultant to WRAIR) suggested that the Maryland malaria program at Jessup might be a suitable venue for the first trial of this promising method in humans. WRAIR agreed to this as a potentially useful sideline to the chemotherapeutic program, and initial vector and irradiation studies commenced under Clyde's direction.

The irradiation of the *P. falciparum*-infected (and soon after, *P. vivax*-infected) *A. stephensi* mosquitoes, prepared in petri dishes by McCarthy, was undertaken enthusiastically by Dr. James E. Robinson and staff in the Department of Radiology. The first trials clarified optimal radiation dosage and the numbers of sporozoites to be injected by the biting mosquitoes. The method called for several massive inoculations of irradiated sporozoites, followed by slide testing against fresh sporozoites by the immunized person's serum to see if agglutination (circumsporozoite precipitation reaction) occurred. Finally, the volunteers were exposed to fresh sporozoites inoculated by nonirradiated mosquitos, to see if malaria developed despite the immunization. Unprotected control volunteers (including the project director who suffered both *falciparum* and *vivax* episodes) were employed in parallel to confirm the infectivity of the fresh sporozoites, which they all did.

After some setbacks, one volunteer became solidly immunized against repeated challenges by infective sporozoites of heterologous strains of *P. falciparum* collected around the world, and soon afterwards more volunteers became protected against both *falciparum* and *vivax* sporozoite challenges. The results, published in 1973 with the expeditious assistance of Harry Most, indicated that sporozoite immunity was species specific but not strain specific, and was stage specific in that it did not protect against blood-induced infections.[9-12]

The malaria program at Jessup closed in the mid-1970s, to be reactivated within the Medical Department's Center for Vaccine Development directed by Dr. Myron M. Levine, who had assisted clinically with the original program at Jessup. The renewed studies took advantage of many advances in technique since the original work and centered on immunization against sporozoites. Following a reprise of the irradiation method of live sporozoites, synthetic and recombinant candidate vaccines were tested in Phase I (dosage tolerance and immunogenicity) and Phase II (protection against challenge) under the direction of Drs. Deirdre E. Herrington and Robert Edelman, with Dr. Jonathan Davis in charge of the mosquito insectary and parasite culture facilities. David Clyde, retiring to Baltimore after several years as Senior Malariologist with WHO in Southeast Asia, rejoined the program in 1985.

REFERENCES

1. McCarthy VC, Clyde DF. Influence of sulfalene upon gametocytogenesis of *Plasmodium falciparum* and subsequent infection patterns in *Anopheles stephensi*. Exp Parasitol 1973;33:73–78.

2. McCarthy VC, Clyde DR. Comparative efficiency of *Anopheles stephensi* and *Anopheles gambiae* as vectors of drug-resistant *Plasmodium falciparum* from Thailand. Am J Trop Med Hyg 1974;23:313.

3. McCarthy VC, Clyde DF, Woodward WE. *Plasmodium falciparum*: Responses of a semi-immune individual to homologous and heterologous challenges, and non-infectivity of gametocytes in *Anopheles stephensi*. Am J Trop Med Hyg 1978;27:6–8.

4. The studies were reported in several papers by D.F. Clyde, and co-authored variously by V.C. McCarthy, and staff of the Division of Infectious Diseases, namely, R.B. Hornick, H.L. DuPont, R.M. Miller, A.T. Dawkins, Jr., R.H. Gilman, A.R. Schwartz, M.M. Levine, and C.C. Rebert: (a) Diformyl diaminodiphenyl sulfone (DFD). Milit Med 1970; 135:527–536; (b) DFD with DDS and chloroquine. Milit Med 1971; 136:836–841; (c) DFD with pyrimethamine. Milit Med 1973;138: 418–421; (d) Sulfalene and trimethoprim. Am J Trop Med Hyg 1971; 20:804–810; (e) Tetracyclines. J Trop Med Hyg 1971;74:238–242; (f) WR33063 and WR30090. Antimicrob. Agents Chemother 1973;3: 220–223; (g) RC-12. Trans R Soc Trop Med Hyg 1974;68:167–178;

(h) Clindamycin. Am J Trop Med Hyg 1975;24:369–370; (i) Mefloquine. Antimicrob Agents Chemother 1976;9:384–386.

5. These studies were reported in papers by D.F. Clyde, and co-authored variously by V.C. McCarthy, R.B. Hornick, H.L. DuPont, W.E. Woodward, A.T. Dawkins, Jr., G.G. Heiner, R.M. Miller, S.I. Music, and R.H. Gilman. The geographical sources of the parasites were these: (a) Thailand & Western Malaysia: Milt Med 1969;134:787–794; (b) Western Malaysia: Trans R Soc Trop Med Hyg 1970;64:834–838; (c) Vietnam: JAMA 1970;213:2041–2045; Am J Trop Med Hyg 1971; 10:1–105; (d) Philippines: J Trop Med Hyg 1971;74:101–105; (e) Burma: J Trop Med Hyg 1973;76:54–60; (f) Sabah: J Trop Med Hyg 1973;76: 226–230; (g) Solomon Islands: J Trop Med Hyg 1974;77:9–12; (h) Indonesia (Irian Jaya): J Trop Med Hyg 1976;79:38–41.

6. Clyde DF. Some characteristics of *Plasmodium vivax* from Vietnam. Proc Helminth Soc Wash 1972;39:70–74.

7. Miller LH, Mason SJ, Clyde DF, McGinnis MH. The resistance factor to *Plasmodium vivax* in Blacks: the Duffy-blood-group genotype, FyFy. N Engl J Med 1976;295:302–304.

8. Clyde DF, McCarthy VC. Radical cure of Chesson strain vivax malaria in man by 7, not 14, days of treatment with primaquine. Am J Trop Med Hyg 1977;26:562–563.

9. Clyde DF, Most H, McCarthy VC, Vanderberg JP. Immunization of man against sporozoite-induced falciparum malaria. Am J Med Sci 1973;226:169–177.

10. Clyde DF, McCarthy VC, Miller RM, Hornick RB. Specificity of protection of man immunized against sporozoite-induced *falciparum* malaria. Am J Med Sci 1973;226:398–403.

11. Clyde DF, McCarthy VC, Miller RM, Woodward WE. Immunization of man against *falciparum* and *vivax* malaria by use of attenuated sporozoites. Am J Trop Med Hyg 1975;24:397–401.

12. McCarthy VC, Clyde DF. *Plasmodium vivax*: Correlation of circumsporozoite precipitation (CSP) reaction with sporozoite-induced protective immunity in man. Exp Parasitol 1977;41:167–171.

17

MALARIA STUDIES AT THE UNIVERSITY OF MARYLAND, 1986–1996

Robert Edelman, M.D.

RATIONALE FOR THE DEVELOPMENT OF MALARIA VACCINES

To better appreciate the contribution of University of Maryland investigators to malaria research, one should be familiar with the status of malaria worldwide. In the 1970s and 1980s, malaria throughout the world began to spin out of control. The widespread resistance of *Anopheles* mosquitoes to insecticides, and the increasing prevalence of chloroquine-resistant strains of *Plasmodium falciparum* in tropical countries, crippled malaria control programs and created a crisis in the clinical therapy of malaria and its prophylaxis. These facts created an urgent need for alternative ways to control malaria. One innovative approach involved the development of malaria vaccines. Potential points of attack included the stimulation of immunity against sporozoites, asexual erythrocytic stages, and sexual stages.

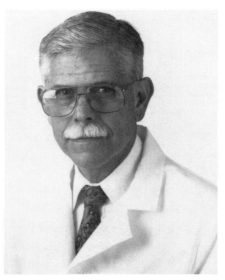

Robert Edelman, M.D.

EARLY IMMUNOPROPHYLACTIC
TRIALS AGAINST EXPERIMENTAL MALARIA

University of Maryland investigators have played a leading role in the effort to develop malaria vaccines. In the early 1970s, a team at the University of Maryland headed by Dr. David Clyde immunized volunteers using x-irradiated, *Plasmodium*-infected mosquitoes to deliver viable, but attenuated sporozoites. After hundreds of such bites, significant protection was elicited against malaria transmitted by the bite of mosquitoes infected with fully virulent *Plasmodium*.[1,2] The demonstration that specific immunity against sporozoite-transmitted malaria could be induced in humans provided much of the critical impetus for research on sporozoite-induced immune mechanisms and vaccine development. It should be noted that for a number of years Dr. Clyde's intriguing observations had little practical application. The protective antigens of *Plasmodium* were largely unknown in the 1970s. Even if protective antigens were known, we had no way to produce them in sufficient quantity to prepare a vaccine for clinical studies in humans. However, major developments in the early 1980s dramatically improved the outlook for malaria vaccines. First, Dr. Ruth Nussenzweig's molecular parasitology group at New York University (NYU) found that antibodies to a simple, repetitive immunodominant sequence on the surface of malaria sporozoites, called the circumsporozoite (CS) protein, protected mice against rodent malaria. Second, the notable advances in biotechnology, including recombinant DNA techniques, peptide synthesis, and use of monoclonal antibodies were applied to basic malaria vaccine research. These seminal discoveries paved the way for the first generation of vaccine candidates.

OPERATION OF A FACILITY FOR STUDY OF MALARIA VACCINES IN VOLUNTEERS

In preparation for the expected onslaught of promising vaccine candidates emanating from the malaria laboratories of the world, the National Institutes of Health (NIH) awarded a five-year contract in 1986 to Dr. Myron M. Levine, Director of the Center for Vaccine Development (CVD). Dr. Levine was funded to operate a facility for the study of malaria vaccines in volunteers. Support was also obtained from the U.S. Agency for International Development, private foundations, and industrial sponsors. To operate this facility, Levine asked Dr. Deirdre Herrington, Assistant Professor of Medicine, to design clinical procedures to safely challenge healthy adult volunteers with laboratory-reared and infected mosquitoes. Dr. David Clyde, who retired to Baltimore after several years as Senior Malariologist with the World Health Organization (WHO) in Southeast Asia, helped conduct the malaria challenge trials. Dr. Robert Edelman assumed responsibility for the clinical trials in 1992, after Dr. Herrington left the University of Maryland. Dr. Levine recruited Dr. James Murphy, Assistant Professor of Microbiology at UMAB, and Dr. Jonathan Davis, a postdoctoral fellow trained in medical entomology, to establish a *Plasmodium* culture laboratory and mosquito insectary to propagate and infect the *Anopheles* vector. Drs. Genevieve Losonsky and Marcelo Sztein conducted some of the immunologic assays at the CVD, but collaborated with Dr. Elizabeth Nardin at NYU, Dr. Dan Gordon at Walter Reed Army Institute of Research (WRAIR), and Dr. Steve Hoffman at the Naval Medical Research Institute, Bethesda, who ran more specialized immunologic assays. Several investigators working in industry kindly supplied unique malarial antigens for assay. The

CVD team worked in parallel with Dr. Jeff Chulay and the malaria vaccine unit at WRAIR, who in 1986 demonstrated that it was possible to infect humans with culture-grown *P. falciparum* transmitted by laboratory-reared mosquitoes. The success of gametocyte cultures eliminated the need for unpredictable human gametocyte donors to obtain sporozoite-infected mosquitoes for challenging immunized volunteers.

CLINICAL TRIALS OF FIRST-GENERATION MALARIA VACCINES

In 1987, the first two malaria vaccines were tested in humans. One of these vaccines was tested at the Walter Reed Army Institute of Research,[3] and the other at the CVD.[4] The army studied a recombinant protein containing 32 repeats of the immunodominant epitope of the CS protein of *P. falciparum* which was purified after expression in *Escherichia coli*. The CVD tested a vaccine prepared by the Hoffmann-La Roche Company in collaboration with Dr. Nussenzweig's group, including Dr. Elizabeth Nardin. This vaccine consisted of the 12-amino-acid synthetic peptide, representing the immunodominant epitope of the *P. falciparum* CS protein conjugated to tetanus toxoid as a carrier protein and adsorbed to aluminum adjuvant. The peptide made medical history, because it was the first fully synthetic protein vaccine ever tested in man. Unhappily, these two vaccines induced only modest levels of antisporozoite antibodies and protected only two of 13 individuals. Nevertheless, the two trials did confirm that at least some humans could be protected by CS subunit protein vaccines. The trials provided the framework for further development and testing of more immunogenic sporozoite vaccines.

Although the CVD was contracted by the NIH to test two vaccines a year between 1986 and 1991, only four subunit vaccines in fact became available from the international malaria network of government and industrial laboratories. The first quasi-successful vaccine tested in 1987[4] was followed by CVD trials of 1) a *P. vivax* recombinant CS protein developed by the Chiron corporation, which was expressed in yeast and adsorbed to alum,[5] and 2) a *P. falciparum* recombinant CS protein developed by MicroGeneSys, Inc., which was expressed in a baculovirus expression vector in insect cells and adsorbed to alum.[6] The antibody response to these two CS subunit proteins adjuvanted with alum was disappointing. As a consequence, a putatively improved CS vaccine was tested in collaboration with Dr. Steve Hoffman at the Naval Medical Research Institute, Bethesda, Maryland.[7] This vaccine candidate, developed by SmithKline Beecham Pharmaceuticals, was a *P. falciparum* recombinant CS protein conjugated to a nonstructural protein of influenza A virus, and expressed in *E. coli.* The vaccine was combined with an experimental adjuvant developed by Ribi Immunochem Research, Inc., consisting of monophosphoryl lipid A, a cell wall skeleton of mycobacteria, and squalane oil. However, only four of 11 volunteers developed high antisporozoite titers despite the powerful adjuvant, and only two of these volunteers were protected against experimental malaria challenge.

CVD investigators sought to develop more robust malaria vaccines by an alternate approach. Under the leadership of Drs. Levine and David Hone, the CS protein was expressed in a living "carrier vaccine," namely, attenuated *Salmonella typhi.* This organism grows intracellularly and is known to stimulate potent cell-mediated immune responses.[8] Although the expression of anti-recombinant CS protein immunity was modest in Salmonella-immunized volunteers, the study provided a benchmark for improved living carrier vaccines, encoding and expressing other malaria antigens.

STUDIES OF THE HUMAN
IMMUNE RESPONSE TO MALARIA

From such disappointing vaccine trials came the recognition that the malaria parasite is an incredibly complex and devious opponent, and that we know relatively little about the protective immune mechanisms in man and what antigens provide protection. This realization created an urgent need for an in-depth reinvestigation of the human immune response associated with protection against sporozoite challenge. We therefore immunized three medical students who volunteered to be bitten by irradiated, *P. falciparum*-infected mosquitoes, using a methodology similar to that used 20 years before by Clyde et al.[1,2] We attempted to characterize the humoral and cellular immune responses of individuals protected by irradiated sporozoites using modern immunologic assays, to define whether the responses were directed against

sporozoite or liver stages, and to define the protective antigens.[9,10] The results of the studies were somewhat disappointing,
in that no consistent immunologic response or protective malarial antigens were identified. However, our studies did set a new
standard for durable sterile immunity against experimental *P. falciparum* malaria, when we discovered one immunized volunteer
who resisted challenge for at least nine months.[10] This fact encouraged investigators sorely in need of a morale boost, and provided a plausible target for future subunit vaccines.

The study of cytokines and their roles in the protective and
pathologic responses to malaria in vaccinees and nonimmunes
was particularly noteworthy.[11,12] The study by Harpaz et al.[11] was
the first prospective analysis of serum cytokine networks in vivo
in humans during the evolution of an infectious process such as
malaria. The study was also the first to compare cytokines in immune and nonimmune individuals during the evolution of the
protective immune response. Growing out of the vaccine trials
was unique information about the immunologic phenomenon of
epitopic suppression.[13] Such studies, conducted in Venezuelans
and Marylanders, demonstrated for the first time in humans that
prior immunity to a carrier protein (in this case, tetanus toxoid)
can suppress the human immune response to a low dose of a
conjugated vaccine (in this case, CS protein coupled to tetanus
toxoid).

REFINEMENT OF EXPERIMENTAL
MALARIA CHALLENGE MODEL IN
VOLUNTEERS AND MOSQUITOES

The need to test the efficacy of these vaccines stimulated the development of a challenge model of *P. falciparum* infection in volunteers inoculated by the bites of infected mosquitoes. The availability of a culture system for *P. falciparum* provided the
mechanism for creating a convenient source of infected mosquitoes capable of transmitting malaria. Together, 45 healthy adult
Maryland volunteers were challenged via the bite of *Anopheles
stephensi* mosquitoes infected with fully virulent *P. falciparum*
sporozoites, and four volunteers were challenged via bites of *A.
stephensi* infected with *Plasmodium vivax* . One hundred percent
of volunteers bitten by five infected mosquitoes were infected,
testifying to the reproducibility of this challenge model. Careful

screening of blood smears for malaria every day enabled a diagnosis to be made before the onset of symptoms in many nonprotected individuals. The experimental challenge system proved to be safe and reproducible. The model provided a rapid, convenient, and relatively inexpensive test of protective efficacy not dependent on vaccine field trials conducted in malaria-endemic countries. Moreover, the volunteer model provided valuable insights into the dynamics of the interaction between the human host and parasite.[14–19]

In addition, the volunteer model provided valuable insights into the dynamics of the interaction between the mosquito host and parasite.[20–27] Particularly noteworthy were the novel *Plasmodium* experiments in mosquitoes that explored the effect of human antisera on *Plasmodium* development and transmission to mice, and on the modulation of *Plasmodium* by antibiotics. Most mosquito experiments were performed in close collaboration with Dr. John Beier's group at the Johns Hopkins School of Hygiene and Public Health.

The failure of the first-generation CS protein subunit malaria vaccines sapped the resources of many industrial, academic, and government agencies and produced the hiatus of clinical malaria research at the CVD between 1994 and 1996. The field is now developing its second wind and starting afresh. Now emphasized are the development and testing of more immunogenic CS vaccines, and multi-antigen erythocytic stage subunit vaccines. During this hiatus, Dr. Edelman helped to guide preclinical development of one promising CS vaccine candidate scheduled for Phase I and II trial at the CVD in 1997.

REFERENCES

1. Clyde DF, McCarthy VC, Miller RM, Hornick RB. Specificity of protection of man immunized against sporozoite-induced *falciparum* malaria. Am J Med Sci 1973;226:398–403.

2. Clyde DF, McCarthy VC, Miller RM, Woodward WE. Immunization of man against *falciparum* and *vivax* malaria by use of attenuated sporozoites. Am J Trop Med Hyg 1975;24:397–401.

3. Ballou WR, Hoffman SL, Sherwood JA, Hollingdale MR, Neva FA, Hockmeyer WT, Gordon DM, Schneider I, Wirtz RA, Young SF, Wasserman GF, Reeve P, Diggs CL, Chulay JD. Safety and efficacy of a recombinant DNA plasmodium falciparum sporozoite vaccine. Lancet 1987;i:1277–1281.

4. Herrington DA, Clyde DF, Losonsky GL, Cortesia M, Murphy JR, Davis J, Baqar S, Felix AM, Heimer EP, Gillesen D, Nardin EH, Nussenzweig RS, Nussenzweig V, Hollingdale MR, Levine MM. Safety and immunogenicity in man of a synthetic peptide malaria vaccine against *Plasmodium falciparum* sporozoites. Nature 1987;328:257–259.

5. Herrington DA, Nardin EH, Losonsky G, Barthurst IC, Barr PJ, Hollingdale MR, Edelman R, Levine MM. Safety and immunogenicity of a recombinant sporozoite malaria vaccine against *Plasmodium vivax*. Am J Trop Med Hyg 1991;45:695–701.

6. Herrington DA, Losonsky GA, Smith G, Volvovitz F, Cochran M, Jackson K, Hoffman SL, Gordon DM, Levine MM, Edelman R. Safety and immunogenicity in volunteers of a recombinant *Plasmodium falciparum* circumsporozoite protein malaria vaccine produced in Lepidopteran cells. Vaccine 1992;10:841–846.

7. Hoffman SL, Edelman R, Bryan J, Schneider I, Davis J, Sedegah M, Gordon D, Church P, Gross M, Silverman C, Hollingdale M, Clyde D, Sztein M, Losonsky G, Paparello S, Jones TR. Safety, immunogenicity, and efficacy of malaria sporozoite vaccine administered with monophosphoryl lipid A, cell wall skeleton of mycobacteria and squalane. Am J Trop Med Hyg 1994;51:603–612.

8. Gonzalez C, Hone D, Noriega F, Tacket CO, Davis JR, Losonsky G, Nataro JP, Hoffman S, Malik A, Nardin E, Sztein MB, Heppner DG, Fouts Tr, Isibasi A, Levine MM. *Salmonella typhi* strain CVD 908 expressing the circumsporozoite protein of *Plasmodium falciparum*: Strain construction, safety and immunogenicity. J Infect Dis 1994;169: 927–931.

9. Herrington D, Davis J, Nardin E, Beier M, Cortese J, Eddy H, Losonsky G, Hollingdale M, Sztein M, Levine MM, Nussenzweig RS, Clyde D, Edelman R. Successful immunization of humans with irradiated malaria sporozoites: Humoral and cellular responses of the protected vaccinees. Am J Trop Med Hyg 1991;45:539–547.

10. Edelman R, Hoffman SL, Davis JR, Belier M, Sztein MB, Losonsky G, Herrington DA, Eddy HA, Hollingdale MR, Gordon DM, Clyde DF. Long-term persistence of sterile immunity in a volunteer immunized with X-irradiated *Plasmodium falciparum*. J Infect Dis 1993;168: 1066–1070.

11. Harpaz R, Edelman R, Wasserman SS, Levine MM, Davis JR, Sztein MB. Serum cytokine profiles in experimental human malaria. Relationship to protection and disease course following challenge. J Clin Invest 1992;90:515–523.

12. Brown AE, Herrington DA, Webster HK, Clyde DF, Sztein MB, Davis JR, Beier MS, Edelman R. Urinary neopterin in volunteers experi-

mentally infected with *Plasmodium falciparum*. Trans R Soc Trop Med Hyg 1992;86:134–136.

13. DiJohn D, Torres JR, Murillo J, Herrington DA, Wasserman SS, Cortesia MJ, Losonsky GA, Sturcher D, Levine MM. Effect of priming with carrier on response to conjugate vaccine. Lancet 1989; 1415–1418.

14. Herrington DA, Clyde DF, Murphy JR, Baqar S, Levine MM, Rosario V, Hollindale MR. A model for *Plasmodium falciparum* sporozoite challenge and very early therapy of parasitaemia for efficacy studies of sporozoite vaccines. Trop Geog Med 1988;10:124–127.

15. Davis JR, Murphy JR, Bazar S, Clyde DF, Herrington DA, Levine MM. Estimate of anti-*Plasmodium falciparum* sporozoite activity in humans vaccinated with synthetic circumsporozoite protein (NANP)$_3$. Trans R Soc Trop Med Hyg 1989;83:748–750.

16. Murphy JR, Baqar S, Davis JR, Herrington DA, Clyde DF. Evidence for a 6.5-day minimum exoerythrocytic cycle for *Plasmodium falciparum* in humans and confirmation that immunization with a synthetic peptide representative of a region of the circumsporozoite protein retards infection. J Clin Micro 1989;27:1434–1437.

17. Murphy JR, Clyde DF, Herrington DA, Baqar S, Davis JR, Palmer K, Cortese J. Continuation of chloroquine-susceptible *Plasmodium falciparum* parasitemia in volunteers receiving chloroquine therapy. Antimicrob Agents Chemother 1990;34:676–679.

18. Davis JR. Laboratory methods for the conduct of experimental malaria challenge of volunteers. Vaccine 1994;12:321–327.

19. Church LWP, Bryan JP, Gordon DM, Edelman R, Fries L, Davis JR, Herrington DA, Clyde DF, Shmuklarsky MJ, Schneider I, McGovern TW, Chulay JD, Ballou RW, Hoffman SL. Clinical manifestations of *Plasmodium falciparum* malaria experimentally induced by mosquito challenge. J Infect Dis 1997;175:915–920.

20. Davis Jr, Murphy JR, Clyde DF, Baqar S, Cochrane AH, Zavala F, Nussenzweig RS. Estimate of *Plasmodium falciparum* sporozoite content of *Anopheles stephensi* used to challenge human volunteers. Am J Trop Med Hyg 1989;40:128–130.

21. Beier JC, Davis JR, Vaughan JA, Noden BH, Beier MS. Quantitation of *Plasmodium falciparum* sporozoites transmitted in vitro by experimentally infected *Anopheles gambiae* and *Anopheles stephensi*. Am J Trop Med Hyg 1991;44:564–570.

22. Davis JR, Cortese JF, Herrington DA, Murphy JR, Clyde DF, Thomas AW, Baqar S, Cochran MA, Thanassi J, Levine MM. *Plasmodium falciparum*: in vitro characterization and human infectivity of a cloned line. Exp Parasitol 1992;74:159–168.

23. Beier MS, Davis JR, Pumpuni CB, Noden BH, Beier JC. Ingestion of *Plasmodium falciparum* sporozoites during transmission of anopheline mosquitos. Am J Trop Med Hyg 1992;47:195–200.

24. Beier JC, Beier MS, Vaughan JA, Pumpuni CB, Davis JR, Noden BH. Sporozoite transmission by *Anopheles freeborni* and *Anopheles gambiae* experimentally infected with *Plasmodum falciparum*. J Am Mosq Contr Assoc 1992;8:404–408.

25. Pumpuni CB, Beier MS, Nataro JP, Guers LD, Davis JR. *Plasmodium falciparum:* Inhibition of sporogonic development in *Anopheles stephensi* by gram-negative bacteria. Exp Parasitol 1993;77:195–199.

26. Davis JR, Beier MS, Beier JC, Pumpuni CB, Edelman R, Herrington C, Clyde DF. Effects of ingested human anti-sporozoite sera on *Plasmodium falciparum* sporogony in *Anopheles stephensi*. Am J Trop Med Hyg 1993;49:174–180.

27. Beier MS, Pumpuni CH, Beier JC, Davis JR. Effects of para-aminobenzoic acid, insulin, and gentamicin on *Plasmodium falciparum* development in anopheline mosquitoes (Diptera: Culcicae). J Med Entomol 1994;31:561–565.

18

DIVISION OF INFECTIOUS DISEASES, 1979–1985

Stephen C. Schimpff, M.D.

My introduction to the Division of Infectious Diseases was in 1969 while serving as a clinical associate at the National Cancer Institute's Baltimore Cancer Research Center, then located at the United States Public Health Service Hospital in Baltimore. I was assigned to direct the intensive care unit and to investigate methods for early diagnosis and treatment of septic shock. Shock commonly occurred in aggressively treated patients with advanced cancer and was the most frequent cause of death. With no in-house mentors in infectious diseases, my supervisor, Dr. Arthur Serpick, a Maryland graduate, suggested Drs. Richard B. Hornick and Mor-

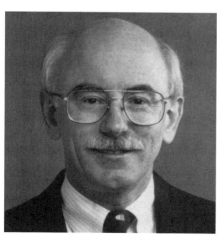

Stephen Schimpff, M.D.

177

ton I. Rapoport as consultants. Thus began a personal "fellowship" in which they
each spent four hours on alternate weeks
as attending physicians over a three-year
period. Later, Dr. Frank M. Calia substi-
tuted once monthly. This stimulating experience began my interactions with the
Division and enduring friendships and
professional relationships.

I made the simple but relevant observation that there was a need to prevent
septic shock by early detection and treatment of Gram-negative bacteremia.

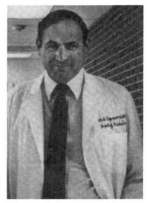

Morton I. Rapoport, M.D.

Nurses and some patients knew that *Pseudomonas aeruginosa*
was the major inciting culprit. The patients whom I interviewed in
my first weeks in Baltimore told me that once infected, patients
were hurried to ICU followed by a trip to
the morgue. I therefore began with a review of the 22 consecutive patients with
P. aeruginosa bacteremia during the previous year. All but one died: 50% were dead
in less than three days after the first positive blood culture. Consistent with early
practice standards, antibiotics were rarely
initiated unless there was specific evidence
of infection other than fever. Our novel
approach initiated specific therapy when
fever occurred in neutropenic patients.
Two investigational agents (carbenicillin
and gentamicin) were available with syn-

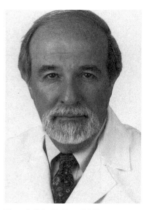

Frank M. Calia, M.D.

ergistic bactericidal activity against *P. aeruginosa*; a protocol was
prepared and approved—although it took four months and some
initial successes to acquire acceptance by my colleagues. The favorable results, reported in the *New England Journal of Medicine*,[1] established a new global standard for care of such patients
and helped launch an academic career.

Another current issue was whether reverse isolation and/or
suppression of alimentary canal flora would reduce infection
rates. There were no reliable data. Viola Mae Young, Ph.D., Director of Microbiology for the Baltimore Cancer Research Cen-

ter, began surveillance cultures of gingiva, nose, axillae, and perianum with semiquantitation and speciation of growth of aerobic bacteria. We cultured leukemia patients on hospitalization and twice weekly thereafter to follow trends in floral changes and to determine the importance of hospital acquisition of potential pathogens. These ill patients, not on antibiotics, rapidly converted predominantly Gram-positive oral flora to Gram-negative rods; both oral and perianal flora often showed within a week or less hospital-acquired flora, especially Gram-negative aerobic bacilli. Antibiotic treatment further hastened these changes and promoted growth of antibiotic-resistant Gram-negatives and yeasts such as *Candida*.[2] Concurrently, we prospectively recorded data on each infected patient over three years. This allowed correlation of the clinical, microbiologic, and surveillance culture data along with levels of granulocytes.[3] Gerald Bodey, M.D., of the National Cancer Institute had previously shown that infections increased in frequency and severity as granulocyte counts declined toward zero. We noted that essentially all Gram-negative bacillary bacteremia occurred only at levels of $<100/\mu l$.[4] These were important implications regarding prevention if alimentary canal flora suppression was contemplated. Obviously, its significance related to those patients with persistent, profound granulocytopenia.

We conducted a randomized, controlled study in adult acute leukemia patients admitted for induction of remission.[5] It involved allocation to laminar air flow room reverse isolation plus use of oral nonabsorbable antibiotics, routine hospital ward care with antibiotics, or ward care alone. Isolation reduced hospital infection acquisition; oral nonabsorbable antibiotics suppressed the alimentary canal flora; and each approach was superior to no action in reducing severe infections including bacteremia. However, there were 1) the psychological implications of isolation, 2) the disagreeable taste of the antibiotics, 3) the cost implications of both approaches, 4) the development of resistant flora among those who received suppression without isolation, and 5) the rapid regrowth of Gram-negative bacteria and subsequent bacteremia when antibiotics were discontinued before return of circulating granulocytes.

Concurrently, Sheldon E. Greisman, M.D., a senior member of the Department of Medicine, had demonstrated the short time or "window" in which antibiotics had to be given before inevitable death would occur in mice with Gram-negative bacteremia.[6] David Johnson, Ph.D., worked with us to develop an animal model of sepsis in the neutropenic rat so that experimental therapies could be evaluated before use in humans.[7]

A particular incident was not only very instructive, but humbling. Dick Hornick came to examine an elderly man with leukemia, no granulocytes, fever, and an *Escherichia coli* bacteremia who poorly responded to combination antibiotic therapy. The site of origin of the infection was elusive. Dr. Hornick asked if I had performed a rectal exam. Upon hearing my embarrassed negative response, he examined the patient with a gloved finger and quietly suggested that I palpate the rectal abscess. Lesson learned. As it turned out, we published a *Lancet* article about two years later[8] documenting the frequency of rectal and perirectal infections in these patients. It prompted a paper in the *Annals of Internal Medicine*[9] which stressed the need for thorough examination to detect sites of origin if critical body areas were emphasized and a limited inflammatory response appreciated. These immune-compromised patients did not manifest the classical signs of pain, redness, swelling, and heat.

Concurrently, senior Department of Medicine members (Drs. Wiswell, Connor, Greisman, and Woodward) gave lectures and made regular teaching rounds in general medicine at the Wyman Park Public Health Service Hospital. By presidential order in the early 1970s, the Public Health Hospitals were programmed to close. Steps were taken by the National Cancer Institute (NCI), NIH, Bethesda, to enlarge or relocate this important center. Dean John W. Moxley III and Dr. George H. Yeager, Hospital Director, appointed an ad hoc committee, with Dr. Woodward as chairman, to encourage recruitment of the Baltimore Cancer Research Center (BCRC) to the Maryland complex. After a series of meetings with Dr. Michael D. Walker, Director of the BCRC, and authorities at NIH, the decision was made for the BCRC to transfer its research unit to the University of Maryland School of Medicine and Hospital in lieu of other options, such as relocating to the Johns Hopkins Medical Institutions or constructing a new facility.

The entire bed and office space of the ninth floor of the South and new North Hospital was transferred to the Baltimore Cancer Research Center, and the Department of Medicine relinquished all of the ninth floor laboratory space in the newly constructed Franck C. Bressler Research Laboratory Building. The BCRC was thus relocated to the University of Maryland Hospital and School of Medicine in 1974. It became a separate program in the School and Medical System as the University of Maryland Cancer Center in 1982 when the NCI withdrew. It was renamed the Marlene and Stewart Greenebaum Cancer Center in 1996 in recognition of a $10 million gift from the Greenebaum family.

When the Baltimore Cancer Research Center moved to the University of Maryland in 1974, relationships with the Division of Infectious Diseases intensified profitably. James Tenney, M.D., hospital epidemiologist, assisted by Harry Oken, M.S., M.D., my student summer fellow, evaluated an unusual species of *Pseudomonas* resistant to most all bactericidal disinfectants. It polluted the complex expensive water sterilization system installed in the Cancer Center's intensive care unit.[10] Working with Dr. Marcia Moody, he evaluated the internal colonization of long-term indwelling vascular catheters. Electron micrographs performed by William Costerton, Ph.D., showed Gram-positive organisms embedded in a glycocalyx along the inner lumen of the catheters. Previously sterile, the catheter developed the glycocalyx formation within six weeks of placement.[11] Remarkably, relatively few patients developed *S. epidermidis* bacteremia from these catheters.

Dr. Harold Standiford was an early and enthusiastic collaborator. He had worked on synergy studies of gram negative bacteria and extended them to the critically ill cancer patients with bacteremia. He then showed that bactericidal levels after antibiotic administration were much better with synergistic combinations, and, together, we demonstrated a survival advantage.

George Drusano, M.D., a former fellow, expanded the study of pharmacokinetics and pharmacodynamics with Hal

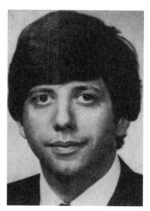

George L. Drusano, M.D.

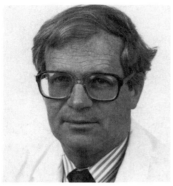
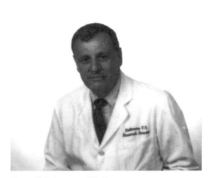

Harold Standiford, M.D.   *David Johnson, Ph.D.*

Standiford and collaborated closely with School of Pharmacy faculty members. Using sophisticated computer modeling techniques, he ably predicted the appropriate dosages and schedules of single agents or combination of agents for maximizing serum concentration, synergistic effect, and serum cidal levels.[12] Drusano and David Johnson used the model to demonstrate the impact of dose fractionation and altered minimal inhibitory concentrations (MICs) on survival of septic rats treated with lomefloxacin. We obtained industry funding applying this model system in evaluating antimicrobial agents for septic neutropenic patients.

Throughout the years, many Division and Cancer Center oncology fellows collaborated with work on infections in cancer patients. James C. Wade, M.D., worked with me and others in the Division and Cancer Center while a fellow in oncology and later as a faculty member. Using molecular epidemiologic methods, *S. epidermidis* bacteremia was shown to originate from alimentary canal flora, not intravascular catheters despite colonization.[13] Well before identification of hepatitis C virus, the high frequency of "nonA-nonB" hepatitis was reported among these patients who received platelet transfusions from multiple donors.[14] The remission time of infection was longer in acute myelocytic leukemia (AML) patients than those not infected. Wade and others also showed that trimethoprim-sulfamethoxazole prophylaxis was found effective in neutropenic patients.[15] Michael Hargadon, a laboratory technologist who later graduated from the University of Maryland School of Dentistry, concurrently showed that oral nonabsorbable antibiotics suppressed anaerobes in addition to aerobes.[16]

Jim Wade initiated a viral surveillance culture system and showed that oral and esophageal infections in AML patients were caused or were preceded by activation and invasion with herpes simplex virus and, occasionally, cytomegalovirus. This prompted use of acyclovir as prophylaxis.

Thomas Walsh, M.D., a former oncology fellow, now at the National Cancer Institute in Bethesda, began studies of fungal infections at the Baltimore Cancer Research Center. With Dave Johnson, he modified the neutropenic animal model for *Candida* and other yeasts.

Jorge Murillo, M.D., worked with Hal Standiford on serum bactericidal levels[17] and skin microbe suppression to prevent axillary lesions during his infectious diseases fellowship.[18] Lillian Love, M.D., an oncology fellow, documented the critical nature of the patient's basic medical status relative to the ultimate outcome of Gram-negative sepsis.[19] Carlos deJongh, M.D., an oncology fellow, reported the importance of synergy in the neutropenic patient.[20] De Jongh, now a leading practitioner in Caracas, Venezuela, also investigated trimethoprim-sulfamethoxazole as prophylaxis.[21] Jai Joshi, M.D., an oncology fellow and then faculty member, evaluated colonization resistance and reported that some antibiotic combinations did not adversely affect alimentary anaerobes[22] and resulted in fewer subsequent infections than did combinations that failed to suppress anaerobes.

Davis Hahn, M.D., now an oncologist in Baltimore, evaluated the use of portable HEPA filters in reducing infections,[4] the use of combination therapy of amikacin and cephalothin,[23] and the value of microbial suppression to reduce infections in leukemia patients.[24] Sheldon Landesman, M.D., now on the faculty of Downstate Medical Center, assisted in the initial studies of empiric therapy with ticarcillin.[25]

Other collaborative studies included the pharmacokinetics of infection in cancer patients and included four pharmacists: Clarence Fortner, M.S., William Grove, M.S., John Bender, M.S. and Rebecca Finley, Pharm.D. They evaluated aminoglycoside administration, the cumulative effects of aminoglycosides on auditory function, the use of single agents rather than combinations for empiric therapy, and other approaches.[26–29]

By the early 1980s, we had a team of many investigators who were contributing to various research activities involving the molecular biology of Gram-negative bacteria, basic and applied microbiology, molecular epidemiology, phamacokinetics and pharmacodynamics, animal models, volunteer and patient Phase I evaluations using serum bactericidal techniques, prospective randomized clinical trials performed at the Cancer Center, and group studies in collaboration with the International Antimicrobial Therapy Study Group. The latter was founded in 1974 by Drs. Jean Klastersky, Harold Gaya, Martin Tattersall, and Stephen Schimpff. This group initially comprised 17 hospital groups in Europe and North America; it later included Australia and the Middle East.[30–33] Other studies at the cancer center were directed toward the epidemiology, prevention, and early diagnosis of viral infections (notably herpes[3,34,35] and hepatitis viruses) and fungal infections (notably *Candida* and *Aspergillus*).[36–38]

In 1979, upon the departure of Richard B. Hornick, M.D., for Rochester, New York, Dr. Woodward asked me to head the Division of Infectious Diseases for the department. After National Cancer Institute approval, I accepted this added and exciting role.

John W. Warren, M.D., joined the Division in 1977 and worked on catheter-related urinary tract infections which included: classical microbiology (bacterial persistence, association with fever, colonization resistance); molecular biology (bacterial adhesions, genetics of urease production), immunology (humoral and cell-mediated response to Tamm-Horsfall protein); pathology (semi-quantitation of renal interstitial lymphocytes and fibrosis and immunochemical staining of Tamm-Horsfall protein); epidemiology (morbidity and mortality of long-term catheter use, risk factors of acute pyelonephritis and fever, prevalence of catheter use in a random sample of Maryland nursing homes); and clinical trials (catheter irrigation, intermittent catheterization, female external collection devices). This research was initially funded by the pharmaceutical industry, followed by an NIH R01 grant and a long-term program project grant extending over 15 years to the year 2000. Warren founded the Division's Antimicrobial Study Group which, from 1979 through 1985, recruited pharmaceutical grants exceeding $1.0 million. This work embraced clinical trials and molecular aspects of antimicrobial action, resistance, and synergy.

Harold Standiford joined the Division in 1971, recruited by Frank Calia and Mort Rapoport, respective heads of Infectious Diseases and the Medical Service at the Baltimore Veterans Administration Hospital. The Veterans Administration converted the Tuberculosis Hospital to an acute care facility in 1968. Standiford soon obtained a Veterans Administration merit review grant. With this grant, studies on antimicrobial combinations and synergy were extended and revealed the high level of aminoglycoside resistance for enterococci and lack of penicillin-aminoglycoside synergy. This grant permitted collaborative research at the Cancer Center, including the potential of studying newer antimicrobial agents for possible use in granulocytopenic infected cancer patients. One such volunteer study compared the pharmacokinetics and serum bactericidal activity of imipenem, compared to standard combination therapy. This led to a large clinical trial to determine its clinical effectiveness. This trial served as a prototype for evaluating antimicrobial regimens before general application. Standiford's work personified the Division's historical record of patient care, teaching, and research.

The vaccine testing program began originally on the hospital medical wards, followed by volunteer studies in prison inmates at the Maryland House of Correction in full collaboration with the Department of Defense investigators at WRAIR and Ft. Detrick. In the 1970s, Drs. Woodward and Hornick began an organized volunteer program in special units of the Hospital. Dr. Myron M. Levine, who had just completed his training at the London School of Hygiene, returned to Maryland and began organization of the Center for Vaccine Development. Levine applied his skills and enthusiasm to make this a continually effective unit as measured by grants, contracts, and research productivity. In 1979, when I became Division Head, the Center operated a 22-bed volunteer ward in University Hospital with laboratory facilities in the old Bressler Research Building. The Division had established an enviable record of vaccine trials supported by long-term contracts from the NIH, CDC, WHO, and PAHO. In 1979 and early 1980s, outstanding investigators were recruited for work on vaccine development.

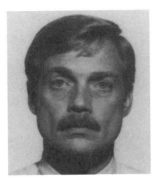

Robert E. Black, M.D.

Robert E. Black, M.D., M.P.H., a former fellow in infectious diseases at UCLA, was also an Epidemiologic Intelligence Service (EIS) officer for the CDC, Atlanta, and a research fellow at the Cholera Research Laboratory in Dacca, Bangladesh. He was appointed Assistant Professor of Medicine and Chief of the Epidemiology Section of the Center for Vaccine Development. He published data of his two years' experience with diarrheal diseases in Dacca and initiated new studies in Baltimore. In Santiago, Chile, he continued and extended the unit's work on typhoid fever vaccine (Ty 21a *S. typhi*) and epidemiologic observations. In Peru, he established collaboration with the Nutrition Research Institute. With investigators at the Peruvian Peruana Heredia University, objective studies were made on the epidemiology of diarrhea and typhoid fever. With Dr. Bradley Sack of the School of Public Health at Hopkins, he studied *Shigella* infections and typhoid fever under a NIH grant. By 1982, he was promoted to Associate Professor and was then a subcommittee member on nutrition and diarrheal disease control for the National Academy of Sciences (NAS). In 1985, he became Professor and Chairman of the Department of International Health at the Johns Hopkins University School of Hygiene and Public Health.

Mary Lou Clements, M.D., M.P.H., formerly Assistant Professor of Medicine at Johns Hopkins, was earlier a special epidemiologist of the WHO Smallpox Eradication Program in India. She came to Maryland in 1980 to be Chief of the Clinical Studies Section of the Center for Vaccine Development. She coordinated outpatient/inpatient volunteer evaluations of the safety, immunogenicity, and efficacy of vaccines against experimental challenge, particularly for influenza and Rocky Mountain spotted fever (RMSF). Her work embraced treatment and management of *Escherichia coli, Campylobacter*, and *Shigella*. Clements attended on the Infectious Diseases, General Medicine Services, and the Traveler's Clinic. In 1985, she returned to Hopkins as Associate Professor in the Department of International Health at the School of Hygiene and Public Health. She became Director of

Vaccine Development at the School in 1986. Her research embraced critical development, safety, and controlled field-testing of new vaccines in large population groups; she was a recognized national authority. Tragically, on September 9, 1998, she, along with her husband, Dr. Jonathan Mann, died in an air accident near Nova Scotia while they were enroute to Geneva to help plan an international strategy against AIDS.

Roy Robins-Browne, M.D., Ph.D., a visiting research fellow in the Center for Vaccine Development in 1979, was formerly registrar, microbiologist, and senior microbiologist at the School of Pathology and South African Institute for Medical Research in Johannesburg. He investigated pathogenesis of diarrhea caused by enteropathogenic *E. coli*, the efficacy of *Lactobacillus* preparations for the prevention and treatment of traveler's diarrhea, and development of serologic assays for cholera. In 1980, he was named Professor and Head of the Department of Microbiology in Melbourne, Australia. He returned for an eight-month sabbatical in 1986 and worked with Glenn Morris on the molecular pathogenesis of infections with *Yersinia enterocolitica*.

Dr. David R. Nalin, an outstanding clinical physiologist, studied cholera and other diarrheal diseases at the Cholera Research Laboratory in Dacca, Bangladesh. He came to Maryland in 1976, and, in 1978, was made Chief of the Physiology Section of the Center for Vaccine Development. Much was accomplished, including demonstration that *E. coli* caused a toxic, noninvasive type of diarrhea. A new enterotoxin of *E. coli* was identified in a dog intestinal loop model, and hypochlorhydria was shown to be a predisposing factor in the pathogenesis of bacterial pathogens. The relationships

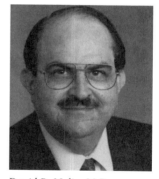

David R. Nalin, M.D.

of antibacterial versus antitoxic immunity were clarified. Nalin and others conducted the first research in Costa Rica to show that oral rehydration and maintenance therapy was effective in rotavirus-infected infants with diarrhea. The first emergency room use of oral therapy for diarrheal diseases was initiated in Costa Rica. He concurrently worked with the World Health Organization (WHO) to design, organize, and supervise studies comparing sucrose with glucose in oral rehydration therapy. In 1979, Nalin was promoted to Associate Professor and named Director of the Pakistan Medical Research Center, Lahore, Pakistan, under Maryland auspices. Studies of suppression of cell-mediated immunity in malaria and reversal after chloroquine therapy followed. Also shown was clustering of malaria in association with high-risk large families. Higher rates of diarrhea and respiratory disease occurred in crowded families with many children. Nalin helped organize the WHO oral therapy training programs and carried out a survey of malaria in a cross section of Karachi and surrounding periurban areas. In 1983, he joined the Merck Research Laboratories and now directs clinical research in the Infectious Diseases Department.

James B. Kaper, Ph.D., joined the Division in 1981, having completed his postdoctoral fellowship at the University of Wash-

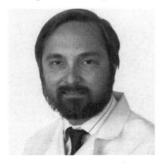

ington in Seattle. He was specifically recruited to develop a program in molecular biology with the intent to create recombinant vaccines for common diarrheal infections, particularly cholera. It was a pleasure to assist Mike Levine in recruiting Jim Kaper, who was arguably the first molelcular biologist and genetic engineer in the School of Medicine. Kaper rapidly set up a very effective lab-

James B. Kaper, M.D., Ph.D.

oratory that has been extremely productive over the years, as attested by a remarkable bibliography. He became full Professor in 1990.

J. Glenn Morris, Jr., M.D., M.P.H., T.M., joined the Division as a fellow in 1982 and the faculty in 1984. He collaborated with Jim Kaper and Mike Levine and, by the Spring of 1984, was awarded a grant for work on *Vibrio vulnificus*. His superb program for evaluation of molecular epidemiology and pathogenesis of bacterial enteric pathogens is a model of its kind. He is Professor of Medicine and directed the newly created Division of Hospital Epidemiology in the Department of Medicine. In January, 2000 he was made Pro-

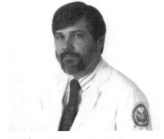

J. Glenn Morris, Jr., M.D.

fessor and Chairman of the Department of Epidemiology and Preventive Medicine.

Under Mike Levine, the Center for Vaccine Development has very successfully obtained grant funding: for example, in 1984, over $3 million in annual grants and contracts came to the Center. Concomitantly, the intramural research program, field studies, and publications were outstanding. Acting on the initial suggestion of Dr. Woodward (letter dated Jan. 29, 1982), in 1984 I recommended to Chairman John A. Kastor, M.D., that the Center for Vaccine Development become the Division of Geographic Medicine within the department. The Division and the Center grew and prospered in the ensuing years.

The Shock Trauma Center was organized by Dr. R Adams

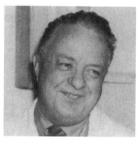

R Adams Cowley, M.D.

Cowley as a four-bed unit within the Department of Surgery in 1963. By 1969, a building financed by Department of Defense funds was built to house the Shock Trauma Center, which then included a 12-bed intensive care unit, three operating rooms, a trauma resuscitation unit, and, over time, a series of step-down units. The Department of Medicine and its Divisions of Infectious Diseases, Nephrology, Cardiology, and Neurology (Neurology became a department in 1964) gave clinical and research support during the developmental stages.

Morton I. Rapoport, M.D., a 1960 graduate, was recruited in 1967 from Ft. Detrick where he conducted fundamental research in infectious diseases.[39–41] Approximately 50% of his time was spent at the Shock Trauma Center evaluating the effect of infection in traumatized patients. An internist physically based in the Shock Trauma Center with focus on infectious diseases and critical care medicine was an innovative concept. This pattern has persisted. Rapoport then headed the Medical Service at the Veterans Administration Hospital beginning in 1971; he was appointed Senior Associate Dean in 1976 and was named Chief Executive Officer of the University of Maryland Medical System in 1982. He is now President and CEO of the system.

I spent three months in the Shock Trauma Center in 1973 and published an early paper on the types of predisposing factors to infection in these multiple traumatized patients.[42]

Ellis Caplan, M.D., became the full-time infectious diseases physician at the Shock Trauma Center in 1976 after 10 years as co-director of the Center for Vaccine Development. Dr. Caplan developed the infectious diseases program in the Trauma Center which included himself, Dr. Manjari Joshi (beginning in 1983), and Dr. Wayne Campbell (beginning in 1989). Together, they defined the

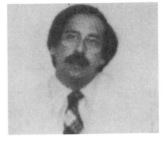

Ellis Caplan, M.D.

types of infections which occur in multiple traumatized patients, developed multiple clinical trials of new antimicrobial agents, evaluated the use of pneumococcal vaccine in splenectomized patients, and established the basic approach to special infectious disease problems in these patients. A unique informative example is that of patients who showed pulmonary infiltrate by chest x-ray, fever, sputum production, and polymorphonuclear leukocytes in the sputum. Yet, when given aggressive chest physical therapy, the "pneumonia" often cleared within a few hours. This indicated that the problem was atelectasis and, hence, no need for antibiotics. Dr. Caplan is recognized nationally and internationally as an authority in the area of infections in the trauma patient.

Frank M. Calia, M.D., came to the Division in 1969 from the Army's program at Ft. Detrick. He was appointed Head of Infectious Diseases at the Loch Raven Veterans Administration Hospital, a position he held until he became Chief of the Medical Service in 1976. Dr. Calia established a laboratory to examine enteric pathogens, particularly vibrios. The role of gastric acid as a defense mechanism was revealed.[43] It was shown that gastric acid is an effective barrier to infections caused by *Vibrio cholerae* and *Salmonella*. This proved to be very helpful in the vaccine protective studies in volunteers. His laboratory was continuously funded by Veterans Administration (VA) merit sources for well over a decade. Calia was Chief of the Medical Service at the VA while I was Head of the Division. In spite of many responsibilities, he attended on a regular basis and never missed weekly infectious diseases conferences which rotated between the Loch Raven Veterans Hospital and University Hospital. For about a year (1975–1976) during these developmental phases of the Division, he directed the entire clinical program.

Merrill J. Snyder, Ph.D., a long-time member of the Division and previous director of the hospital microbiology laboratories, was the Division's prime internal critic. He helped all faculty and fellows with superb manuscript reviews and techniques of presentation. Snyder was an outstanding contributor to the design and analysis of laboratory and clinical studies.

The Division was extremely fortunate to have the unstinting and enthusiastic support of many infectious diseases physicians who practiced in the community. They attended on the wards and regularly participated in weekly clinical and research conference. Among them were Jay S. Goodman, M.D., Professor of Medicine and Chief of Medicine at Mercy Hospital; Ronald Geckler, M.D., Head of Infectious Diseases at Mercy Hospital; the late J.J. Gunning, M.D., Vice President for Medical Affairs at St. Agnes; Jerry Seals, M.D., Chief of Infectious Diseases at Howard County General Hospital; and John McConville, M.D., Head of Infectious Diseases at York Hospital in Pennsylvania. They added depth and breadth to the Division's teaching program. They brought a wealth of experience from their own personal backgrounds and allowed the fellows, residents, and students to hear the perspective of practicing physicians as opposed to academicians. Laboratory capability is critical to the training of fellows and students. Sharon Hansen, Ph.D., director of the microbiology laboratories at the Veterans Hospital was outstanding in her teaching and research projects which evaluated new technologies for the efficient, effective operation of the diagnostic laboratories.

The Division established an excellent educational and training program as a result of outstanding full-time and volunteer faculty, personnel, patient diversity (University Hospital general infectious diseases, the Veterans Administration Hospital infectious diseases program, the Cancer Center, the Shock Trauma Center, the Traveler's Clinic), and faculty enthusiasm for teaching. The infectious diseases rotation was a favorite elective for senior medical students and medical and pediatric residents. Outstanding candidates were attracted to the fellowship program.

The Division offices on the fifth floor of the Bressler Building in 1979 gave the appearance of antiquity, without renovation since the building was constructed in 1933. With support from the Dean's office, we obtained $20,000 from the School of Medi-

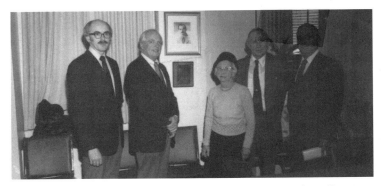

Dedication of McCrumb Conference Room. Left to right: S. Schimpff; J.M. Dennis, Dean; Mrs. Fred R. McCrumb, Sr.; T. Woodward; McCrumb family relative.

cine and, with help from Jack Warren and Carol Schimpff (as a pro bono architect), a frugal but very comfortable renovation of the entire fifth floor was accomplished. It included a conference room named for Fred McCrumb, M.D., a prior director of the Division who died suddenly at age 50. With funds from the Department of Medicine, an ultracentrifuge and scintillation counter were obtained for Jim Kaper, and Cancer Center project funds helped acquire gas liquid chromatography equipment for George Drusano. Proceeds from a Division antibiotic trial helped purchase the first word processor (no small purchase; in those days computer applications were expensive and the word processor cost $10,000); the morale of Eunice Katz, Division Secretary, now Division Administrator, increased dramatically. In 1984, the Division was separated into Infectious Diseases and Geographic Medicine Divisions of the department and moved to new quarters on the ninth floor of the Medical School Teaching Facility. In 1985, I stepped down as Division Head and began a new position as Executive Vice President of the University of Maryland Medical System, and in 1999 CEO of the University of Maryland Medical Center.

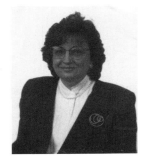

The years 1979–1985 were productive years for the Division, marked by strong research programs, firm teaching, and solid patient care commitments. A list of the Division faculty for those years follows:

Eunice P. Katz
Divisional Administrator

Full Time: Frank M. Calia, M.D., Ellis S. Caplan, M.D., George L. Drusano, M.D., Sharon Hansen, Ph.D., David E. Johnson, Ph.D., Harry L.T. Mobley, M.D., Stephen C. Schimpff, M.D. (Division Head), Merrill J. Snyder, Ph.D., Harold C. Standiford, M.D., James H. Tenney, M.D., John W. Warren, M.D.

Part-time or Volunteer Faculty: Ronald Geckler, M.D., Jay S. Goodman, M.D., J.J. Gunning, M.D., John McConville, M.D., Gerald Seals, M.D.

Fellows: William Anthony, M.D., Chandalekha Banerjee, M.D., Eric Bergquist, M.D., Luis Cisneros, M.D., Dino Delaportas, M.D., Mark Finch, M.D., Brian Fitzpatrick, M.D., Arnold Henson, M.D., Dierdre Herrington, M.D., Preston Holley, M.D., Margaret Hom, M.D., Rima Khabbaz, M.D., James King, M.D., Andrew Krinsky, M.D., Claudio Lanata, M.D., Carlos Lopez, M.D., William B. McNamee, M.D., J. Glenn Morris, M.D., Jorge Murillo, M.D., Dan Perlman, M.D., Guillermo Prada, M.D., Stephen Sears, M.D., John Sixbey, M.D., Steven B. Sotman, M.D., Pablo Vial, M.D., Deborah Weber, M.D.

REFERENCES

1. Schimpff S, Satterlee W, Young VM, Serpick A. Empiric therapy with carbenicillin and gentamicin for febrile patients with cancer and granulocytopenia. N Engl J Med 1971;284:1061–1065.

2. Newman KA, Schimpff SC, Young VM, Wiernik PH. Lessons learned from surveillance cultures from patients with acute nonlymphocytic leukemia: Usefulness for epidemiologic, preventive and therapeutic research. Am J Med 1981;70:423–431.

3. Schimpff S, Serpick A, Block J, Stoler B, Rumack B, Mellin H, Joseph J. Varicella zoster infection in patients with cancer. Ann Intern Med 1972;76:241–254.

4. Schimpff SC, Hahn DM, Brouillet MD, Young VM, Wiernik PH. Infection prevention in acute leukemia. Comparison of basic infection prevention techniques with standard room reverse isolation or with reverse isolation plus added air filtration. Leukemia Res 1978;2:231–240.

5. Schimpff SC, Greene WH, Young VM, Fortner CL, Jepsen L, Cusack N, Block JB, Wiernik PH. Infection prevention in acute nonlymphocytic leukemia. Laminar air flow room reverse isolation and, oral, nonabsorbable antibiotic prophylaxis. Ann Intern Med 1975;82: 351–358.

6. Greisman SE, DuBuy JB, Woodward CL. Experimental gram-negative bacterial sepsis: Prevention of mortality not preventable by antibiotics alone. Infect Immun 1979;25:538–557.

7. Johnson DE, Thompson B. Efficacy of single-agent therapy with azlocillin, ticarcillin, and amikacin and beta-lactam/amikacin combinations for treatment of *Pseudomonas aeruginosa* bacteremia in granulocytopenic rats. Am J Med 1986;80(S5C):53–58.

8. Schimpff SC, Wiernik PH, Block JB. Rectal abscesses in cancer patients. Lancet 1972;ii:844–847.

9. Schimpff S, Young V, Greene W, Vermeulen G, Moody M, Wiernik P. Origin of infection in acute nonlymphocytic leukemia-significance of hospital acquisition of potential pathogens Ann Intern Med 1972;77:707–714.

10. Newman KA, Tenney JH, Oken H, Moody MR, Wharton R, Schimpff SC. Persistent isolation of an unusual *Pseudomonas* sp. from phenolic disinfectant system for laminar air flow rooms. Infect Control 1984;5:219–222.

11. Tenney JH, Moody MR, Newman KA, Schimpff SC, Wade JC, Costerton JW, Reed WH. Adherent micro-organisms on luminal surfaces of long-term intravenous catheters: importance of *Staphylococcus epidermidis* in patients with cancer. Arch Intern Med 1986;146: 1949–1954.

12. Drusano GL, Standiford H, Ryan P, McNamee W, Tatem B, Schimpff S. Correlation of predicted serum bactericidal activities and values measured in volunteers. Eur J Clin Microbiol 1986;5:88–92.

13. Wade JC, Schimpff SC, Newman KA, Wiernik PH. *Staphylococcus epidermidis*: an increasing cause of infection in granulocytopenic patients. Ann Intern Med 1982;97:503–508.

14. Wade JC, Wiernik PH, Schimpff SC, Hoofnagle JH, Schiffer CA. Hepatitis among patients with acute nonlymphocytic leukemia. Ann Intern Med 1983;75:413–422.

15. Wade JC, Schimpff SC, Hargadon MT, Fortner CL, Young VM, Wiernik PH. A comparison of trimethoprim/sulfamethoxazole plus nystatin with gentamicin plus nystatin in the prevention of infections in acute leukemia. N Engl J Med 1981;304:1057–1062.

16. Hargadon MT, Young VM, Schimpff SC, Wade JC, Minah GE. Selective suppression of alimentary tract microbial flora as prophylaxis during granulocytopenia. Antimircrob Agents Chemother 1981;20: 620–624.

17. Murillo J, Standiford HC, Schimpff SC, Tatem BA. Comparison of serum bactericidal activity among three antimicrobial combinations. Antimicrob Agents Chemother 1978;13:992–996.

18. Murillo J, Schimpff SC, Brouillet MD. Axillary lesions in patients with acute leukemia: Evaluation of a preventive program. Cancer 1979;43:1493–1496.

19. Love LJ, Schimpff SC, Schiffer CA, Wiernik PH. Improved prognosis for granulocytopenic patients with gram-negative bacteremia. Am J Med 1980;68:643–648.

20. deJongh CA, Joshi JH, Newman KA, Moody MR, Wharton R, Standiford HC, Schimpff SC. Antibiotic synergism and response in gram-negative bacteremia in granulocytopenic cancer patients. Am J Med 1986;80:96–100.

21. deJongh CA, Wade JC, Finley RS, Joshi JH, Aisner J, Wiernik PH, Schimpff SC. Trimethoprim/sulfamethoxazole versus placebo: a double blind comparison of infection prophylaxis in patients with small cell carcinoma of the lung. J Clin Oncol 1983;1:302–307.

22. Joshi JH, Newman KA, Brown BW, Finley RS, Ruxer RL, Moody MA, Schimpff SC. Double β-lactam regimen compared to an aminoglycoside/β-lactam regimen as empiric antibiotic therapy for febrile granulocytopenic cancer patients. Support Care Cancer 1993;1: 186–194.

23. Hahn DM, Schimpff SC, Young VM, Fortner CL, Standiford HC, Wiernik PH. Amikacin and cephalothin: an empiric regimen for granulocytopenic cancer patients. Antimicrob Agents Chemother 1977; 12:618–624.

24. Hahn DM, Schimpff SC, Fortner CL, Smyth AC, Young VM, Wiernik PH. Infection in acute leukemia patients receiving oral nonabsorbable antibiotics. Antimicrob Agents Chemother 1978;13:958–964.

25. Schimpff SC, Landesman S, Harn DM, Standiford HC, Fortner CL, Young VM, Wiernik PH. Ticarcillin in combination with cephalothin or gentamicin as empiric antibiotic therapy in granulocytopenic cancer patients. Antimicrob Agents Chemother 1976;10:837–844.

26. Bender JF, Schimpff SC, Young VM, Fortner CL, Brouillet MD, Love LJ, Wiernik PH. The role of vancomycin as a component of oral nonabsorbable antibiotics for microbial suppression in leukemic patients. Antimicrob Agents Chemother 1979;15:455–460.

27. Bender JF, Schimpff SC, Young VM, Fortner CL, Love LJ, Brouillet MD, Wiernik PH. A comparative trial of tobramycin versus gentamicin in combination with vancomycin and nystatin for alimentary tract suppression in leukemic patients. Eur J Cancer 1979;15:35–44.

28. Bender FJ, Fortner CL, Schimpff SC, Grove WR, Hahn DM, Love LJ, Wiernik PH. Comparative auditory toxicity of aminoglycoside antibiotics in leukopenic patients. Am J Hosp Pharm 1979;36:1083–1087.

29. Finley RS, Fortner CL, de Jongh CA, Wade JC, Newman KA, Caplan ES, Brittner J, Wiernik PH, Schimpff SC. Comparison of standard versus pharmacokinetically adjusted amikacin dosing in granulocytopenic cancer patients. Antimicrob Agents Chemother 1982;22:193–197.

30. EORTC International Antimicrobial Therapy Project Group (Writing Committee: Schimpff SC, Gaya H, Klastersky J, Tattersall MHN, Zinner SH). Three antibiotic regimens in the treatment of infection in febrile granulocytopenic patients with cancer. J Infect Dis 1978; 137:14–29.

31. EORTC International Antimicrobial Therapy Project Group (Writing Committee: Zinner SH, Gaya H, Glauser MP, Klastersky J, Schimpff SC, Tattersall MHN). Combination of amikacin and carbenicillin with or without cefazolin as empirical therapy of febrile neutropenic patients. J Clin Oncol 1983;1:597–603.

32. EORTC International Antimicrobial Therapy Project Group (Writing Committee: Zinner SH, Schimpff SC, Klastersky J, Gaya H, Glauser M,Tattersall MHN). Trimethoprim-sulfamethoxazole in the prevention of infection in neutropenic patients. J Infect Dis 1984;150: 372–379.

33. EORTC International Antimicrobial Therapy Project Group. Ceftazidine combined with a short or long course amikacin for empirical therapy of gram-negative bacteremia in cancer patients with granulocytopenia. N Engl J Med 1987;317:1692–1698.

34. Schimpff SC, Fortner CL, Greene WH, Wiernik PH. Cytosine arabinoside for localized herpes zoster in patients with cancer: Failure in a controlled trial. J Infect Dis 1974;130:673–676.

35. Ruckdeschel JC, Schimpff SC, Smyth AC, Mardiney MR Jr. Herpes zoster and impaired cell-associated immunity to the varicella-zoster virus in patients with Hodgkin's disease. Am J Med 1977;62:77–85.

36. Aisner J, Schimpff SC, Bennett JE, Young VM, Wiernik PH. Aspergillus infections in cancer patients: Association with fireproofing materials in a new hospital. JAMA 1976;235:411–412.

37. Aisner J, Schimpff SC, Wiernik PH. Treatment of invasive aspergillosis: Relation of early diagnosis and treatment to response. Ann Intern Med 1977;86:539–543.

38. Aisner J, Murillo J, Schimpff SC, Steere AC. Invasive aspergillosis in acute leukemia: Correlation with nose cultures and antibiotic usage. Ann Intern Med 1979;90:4–9.

39. Rapoport MI, Beisel WR. Circadian periodicity of tryptophan metabolism. J Clin Invest 1968;47:934.

40. Beisel WR, Rapoport MI. Adrenocortical function and infectious illness: Part I. N Engl J Med 1969;28:541.

41. Beisel WR, Rapoport MI. Adrenocortical function and infectious illness: Part II. N Engl J Med 1969;28:596.

42. Schimpff SC, Miller R Polakavetz, Hornick R. Infection in the severely traumatized patient. Ann Surg 1974;179:352–357.

43. Calia, FM, Johnson, DE, Wentz, DK, Snyder, MJ, Hornick, RB. In-vitro sensitivity of bacterial enteropathogens to hydrogen-ion. Eleventh Interscience Conference on Antimicrobial agents and Chemotherapy, Atlantic City, New Jersey, October 22, 1971.

19

Vaccine Research: Clinical Trials, Field Trials, and Basic Research, 1970–1997

Myron M. Levine, M.D., D.T.P.H.

THE EPIDEMIOLOGIC
INTELLIGENCE SERVICE YEARS, 1970–1973

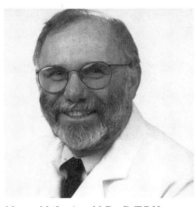

Myron M. Levine, M.D., D.T.P.H.

My original duty assignment in 1970, by the U.S. Public Health Service (PHS), as an Epidemiologic Intelligence Service (EIS) officer, was to the Division of Infectious Diseases of the University of Maryland. Dr. Richard B. Hornick was then the Division Head and, with Dr. Herbert L. DuPont and others, research on *Shigella* vaccines was under evaluation to determine what might prove useful for control of endemic shigellosis in custodial institutions. Col. David Mel in Yugoslavia had reported excellent efficacy results in field studies with streptomycin-dependent attenuated strains of *Shigella* used as live oral vaccines. Dr. Samuel

B. Formal of the Walter Reed Army Institute of Research (WRAIR) had developed a strategy to attenuate wild-type *Shigella*. His *S. flexneri* 2a vaccine generated encouraging results in Phase 2 clinical trials. There was a long-standing close affiliation between the Maryland and WRAIR groups. Beginning in late 1968, epidemic dysentery caused by *S. dysenteriae* 1 (the Shiga bacillus) occurred in several countries in Central America. This became a full-fledged pandemic of Shiga dysentery in 1969 with high mortality and was regarded as a public health emergency. Hence, the focus of *Shigella* vaccine changed to Shiga dysentery vaccines. The Centers for Disease Control (CDC) responded to this problem by altering my official assignment from Baltimore to El Salvador (where there was a CDC field station). The plan of my supervisor at CDC (Dr. Eugene J. Gangarosa, a former faculty member at Maryland) was for me to be responsible for designing and conducting a field trial of a Shiga dysentery vaccine candidate that Dr. Formal had developed (on the assumption that it would prove safe, immunogenic, and protective in preliminary clinical trials in adult volunteers). While administrative procedures were being arranged with the El Salvador government, CDC assigned me to initiate work in Baltimore, rather than Atlanta. Thus, in 1970, I arrived in Baltimore for temporary duty to carry out Phase 1 and 2 studies with Formal's Shiga vaccine candidate, as a preliminary step before moving to Central America.

Because of bureaucratic difficulties, including a delay in obtaining governmental clearance from El Salvador, my presumed temporary duty in Baltimore took shape as a longer term sojourn. Accordingly, with others, clinical research protocols were initiated to test the safety and immunogenicity of candidate *S. dysenteriae* 1 vaccines in adult volunteers at the Maryland House of Correction and to evaluate *S. sonnei* and *S. flexneri* 2a vaccines in children at Rosewood State Hospital in Owings Mills, Maryland. The Division of Infectious Diseases had established excellent relationships with these institutions.

During this period, Dick Hornick warmly welcomed me to the Division. This included paving the way to practice pediatric infectious diseases within the University of Maryland Hospital. I had entered the EIS program in 1970 from Bronx Municipal Hospital Center/Albert Einstein School of Medicine where I had completed a pediatric residency and a short pediatric infectious diseases fellowship under the supervision of Dr. John Robbins (who was Chief of Pediatric Infectious Diseases at Einstein until 1970). In 1971, Dr. Hornick arranged with Dr. Marvin Cornblath, the Chairman of Pediatrics, for me to formalize a pediatric infectious diseases consultation service at the University of Maryland Hospital. Previously there were no full-time pediatric infectious disease consultants. During this same period (early 1971), at the behest of the U.S. Public Health Service, and with the support of Drs. Gangarosa, DuPont, and Hornick and others, two randomized controlled field trials of efficacy of live oral *Shigella* vaccines were initiated in Willowbrook State Hospital in Staten Island, New York and in Sunland Training Center in Lehigh Acres, Florida.

In the early 1970s, the Division of Infectious Diseases was housed in old facilities on the fourth and fifth floors of the Bressler Research Building in 29 South Greene Street (now called the Greene Street Building). There were only a few basic laboratory research activities in the Division. The fundamental studies of Shelly Greisman on the smaller vascular circulation, hemorrhagic, septic shock, and the nature and role of endotoxin gained national and international recognition (see Chapter 13). By contrast, clinical research was thriving and many well-designed and carefully executed clinical protocols were underway. The clinical

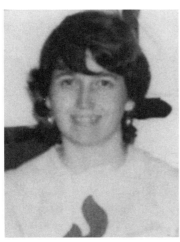 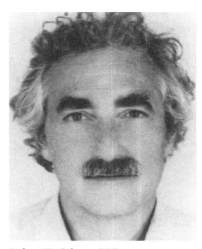

Ronica Kluge, M.D.   *Robert H. Gilman, M.D.*

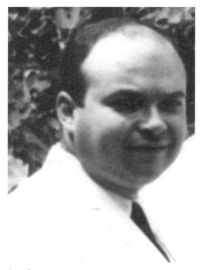

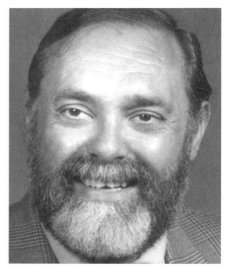

Stanley Music, M.D.   *Richard Cash, M.D.*

orientation included an active teaching program with multiple bright and energetic fellows, including Drs. Donald Pachuta, Ronica Kluge, Robert Gilman, Stanley Music, Richard Cash, Andrew Schwartz, Ellen Wald, John McConville, and Ellis Caplan. The care of patients with infectious disease problems, both inpatient and outpatient, was then a pivotal part of daily activities in the Division. Everyone attended the weekly Monday afternoon clinical infectious diseases conference. Dick Hornick was a popular and inspiring leader. Morale was high, and there was an admirable esprit de corps.

Several major changes occurred in the Division in 1973. Bert DuPont left, having accepted a job to become Director of the Program in Infectious Diseases and Microbiology at the newly founded University of Texas at Houston. Through departmental and medical school channels, Drs. Hornick and Cornblath, respectively, arranged for me to be appointed Assistant Professor of Medicine and Pediatrics in 1972,

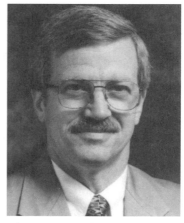

John H. McConville, M.D.

while I was a CDC employee on assignment to the Division. By early 1973, as a consequence of my three years with the Division of Infectious Diseases at Maryland and my association with the CDC and with other investigators in the Division, I gained considerable experience in the evaluation of live oral *Shigella* and typhoid vaccines. This stimulated me to conduct large-scale field trials in endemic areas with some of the most promising vaccine candidates. To explore this concept, in March and April, 1973, as a Pan American Health Organization consultant, I visited six countries in Central and South America to survey possible sites for a field unit to study enteric infections. Peru was the country selected for such a future site, and we submitted a grant request to the Agency for International Development (AID) for support of the unit. In the meantime in 1973, I left the Public Health Service and, with the support of Drs. Hornick and Woodward, I joined the Division of Infectious Diseases on a full-time basis in September. The 1973–1974 academic year was spent at the London School of Tropical Medicine and Hygiene. This experience, coupled with my years at the CDC, made me eligible to sit for the Preventive Medicine Board examination, provided formal training in tropical public health, and prepared me for my expected task of developing a field unit in Peru.

THE CRCVD AND EARLY CVD WITHIN THE DIVISION OF INFECTIOUS DISEASES, 1974–1984

In 1974, relations between the United States and Peru became severely strained, and U.S. AID decided not to fund the grant for the field unit, even though the project was technically approved. In May 1974, Dick Hornick called me in London to explain the drastically altered situation. This was my first sobering introduction to the realities of funding practices in academia. Hornick indicated that the financial situation in the Division was constrained, but that the Division had just been awarded a one-year pilot research contract by the National Institute of Allergy and Infectious Diseases (NIAID) to develop a 10-bed research isolation ward for testing vaccines in community volunteers. Dr. Robert Chanock, Chief of the Laboratory of Infectious Diseases (LID) at NIAID, wanted to explore the feasibility of operating a Research Isolation Unit for testing candidate vaccines from the LID to establish their safety, immunogenicity, and efficacy in inpatient volunteers recruited from the general community. The volunteers were expected to be housed under physical containment for 10–30 days. With the exception of *Mycoplasma pneumoniae*, all the vaccines under development by LID investigators were for viruses including influenza, respiratory syncytial virus, parainfluenza, and rotavirus. An inpatient containment facility was needed, since the principal strategy of LID was to develop attenuated strains of these viruses for administration as live intranasal or oral vaccines. Also, the unit would attempt to conduct experimental challenge studies with wild-type viruses in order to assess, in a preliminary manner, the efficacy of the candidate vaccines. This emphasis on respiratory viruses was a departure from the main focus and strength of Maryland's Division of Infectious Diseases during the previous decade (i.e., bacterial and rickettsial infections). (See Chapter 15 by Dr. Togo regarding studies of influenza, rhinovirus infections, use of vaccines, and the common cold.)

The work scope of this one-year research contract included no laboratory activities whatsoever. The mandate was to establish a containment facility, organize a program to recruit healthy adult volunteers from the general Baltimore community, perform the clinical studies, and collect the clinical specimens which were all to be processed at the LID.

Upon my return to Baltimore in July 1974, with strong support of University Hospital authorities, we began to prepare the containment facility, hire nurses and recruiters, establish standard operating procedures, and arrange administrative policies for the unit. One of our first innovations was to furnish the ward in an ambience that resembled a college dormitory. Since a 10-bed unit allowed only limited clinical data to be generated with a single study, we expanded the ward to 22 beds by simply ordering double-decker bunk beds. This allowed more than double the initial capacity within the same limited space of the original small ward. The first clinical study, a Phase 1 trial of a mycoplasma vaccine, was initiated in October 1974—several months ahead of schedule.

We designated the initial unit the Clinical Research Center for Vaccine Development (CRCVD). After one year of viral vaccine studies, including several influenza virus challenges and collection of specimens for the LID to process, the National Institutes of Health (NIH) graciously awarded us a four-year research contract to support the unit. Although gratified with this program, I personally felt restless, and missed the field work and the opportunity to study the diseases in which I was most interested, namely, bacterial enteric infections like shigellosis, typhoid fever, cholera, and *Escherichia coli* diarrhea. During these first two years, Dr. Ellis Caplan, who worked as a clinical investigator with the CRCVD from 1974 to 1976, provided invaluable assistance and was instrumental, along with others, in helping the CVD to become established.

In August 1975, at the invitation of Dr. Stanley Foster, head of the Smallpox Eradication Program in Bangladesh, I went to Bangladesh for three months to work with the World Health Organization Smallpox Eradication Program. Dr. Ellis Caplan supervised the unit during these several months. While working in the field with the smallpox program, I reflected at length on the previous 12 months of my professional life and contemplated the future, for myself and the unit. On return to Baltimore, I decided to visit the project officer at NIH and attempt to modify drastically the work scope and the scientific focus of the CRCVD. My goal was to expand the unit to include laboratory support for ancillary immunologic and microbiologic studies and modify the work scope to allow Maryland investigator-initiated clinical research protocols on bacterial enteric infections. Another objective was to attract other investigators for work on fundamental aspects of vaccine development. In addition, my impelling desire was to establish collaborative research projects in developing countries where the enteric infections that interested me were rampant. These basic research laboratory efforts and the epidemiologic field activities were conceived to complement and strengthen the clinical research activities. In November 1995, with Dr. Hornick, we visited the late Dr. John Seal at NIH and gained the support of our objectives. John Seal was then Scientific Director of NIAID and project officer for the research contract. He was very supportive and enthusiastic, and stated his belief that these modifications would strengthen the unit and allow the retention of energetic and creative faculty. He agreed to arrange a modification of the contract to include a bacteriology technician and an immunology technician. Although this was only a modest beginning, an important precedent was set. In January 1976, acknowledging this fundamental alteration in the work scope and orientation of the unit, the CRCVD was renamed the Center for Vaccine Development (CVD). This change was made in recognition of the expansion of activities to include laboratory research and epidemiologic field research, all intended to be cornerstones of the Center's expanding mission. Within three years, each of these objectives was achieved.

In early 1976, the first clinical research protocols from Maryland investigators were initiated, which included a safety/immunogenicity trial of an oral and a parenteral cholera vaccine (glutaraldehyde cholera toxin) and pathogenesis and infection-derived immunity studies with selected enterotoxigenic *E. coli* strains.

During 1977, I periodically consulted with the Pan American Health Organization and the U.S. Agency for International Development on limited projects to enhance the use of oral rehydration for treatment of diarrheal dehydration. These projects involved several clinical research trials of infant diarrhea, two microbiologic studies, and design of national diarrheal disease control programs for two countries. This helped establish a network of colleagues and collaborators in many countries in Latin America and several in Africa that would serve the CVD well in years to come as a means to undertake collaboration, with competent investigations in many countries. In 1978, Dr. David Nalin joined the CVD. Previously Nalin had contributed importantly to our knowledge of physiologic abnormalities in cholera patients while in Dacca. He later directed the ICMRT Program in Lahore, 1979–1981 (see Chapter 18). His vast experience in cholera and intestinal physiology, his well-earned international reputation for his significant contributions in development of oral rehydration, his multilingual expertise, and his willingness to work on projects in developing countries for several months at a time made Nalin a vital member of the CVD. One principal focus of clinical research during his years at the CVD was on making oral rehydration a practical therapy. These studies, now recognized as a model of their type through clinical trials in several developing countries, helped optimize oral rehydration of infants with moderate diarrheal dehydration. In the laboratory, his principal investigative interests involved a search on novel enterotoxins in cer-

tain categories of diarrheagenic *E. coli* and evaluation of chiti-
nase in allowing *V. cholerae* to colonize the chitinous exoskeleton
of certain crustacea and zaoplankton.

In 1978, the Pan American Health Organization and the
Ministry of Health of Chile invited me to spend five weeks in
Chile reviewing the epidemiologic problem of endemic typhoid
fever in the metropolitan region of Santiago and to design possible cost-effective interventions. All of November and part of December were spent in Chile working on this fascinating problem,
during which time I became captivated by the country and its
people. My host was Dr. Jose-Manuel Borgoño, Head of the Epidemiology Unit. Upon return to Baltimore, a grant was prepared
to establish an epidemiologic and microbiologic infrastructure in
Santiago. This included studies of the reservoir of infection,
modes of transmission, evaluation of screening methods to identify chronic typhoid carriers, nonsurgical methods to treat carriers, and a large-scale field evaluation of the efficacy of Ty21, a
live oral typhoid vaccine. When this project was funded in 1980,
it became the basis of the Typhoid Fever Control Program in the
Ministry of Health. It was my privilege to be the advisor to this
program throughout its existence until it was disbanded in 1992.
This also marked the start of a continuous presence in Chile of
research activities carried out by the CVD. Thus the goal of establishing a field research unit was achieved. Not only did the
unit in Chile flourish for research on enteric and other infectious
diseases, but it proved to be a fertile site for training infectious
disease (ID) fellows interested in international health. Indeed, as
an increasing number of articles appeared in scientific journals
that described research activities of the CVD, increasing numbers
of superior candidate fellows became attracted to the ID fellowship program at Maryland, in great part influenced by the training opportunities offered by the CVD.

Finally, in the period 1978 to 1980, efforts were initiated to
establish a credible basic science research program in vaccinology
at the CVD. The first step involved organizing an immunology
laboratory capable of assessing serum and intestinal SigA antibodies against enteric pathogens, using the most up-to-date
methods then available (ELISA and Y-1 adrenal cell tissue culture
assays). Also, the latest techniques to detect several bacterial en-

teric pathogens of interest were instituted in the clinical microbiology laboratory.

In 1978, Dr. Roy Robins-Browne came to the CVD from South Africa to spend a sabbatical year. He added a bevy of additional sophisticated microbiologic and biochemical assays such as a method to measure guanylate cyclase activity for detecting biologic activity of *E. coli* heat-stable enterotoxin.

A most important and enduring step taken to initiate a fundamental vaccine development was the recruitment in 1980 of Dr. James B. Kaper as Chief of the Bacterial Genetics Section of the CVD. In 1980, when the era of recombinant DNA technology was in its infancy, this new methodology allowed the CVD to construct a new generation of live oral cholera vaccine strains. These were attenuated by rational and precise genetic manipulation. Within a few years using genetic manipulation, Kaper and his laboratory team constructed the first several prototype attenuated *Vibrio cholerae* O1 vaccine strains. These first engineered vaccine candidates, such as JBK 70 and CVD 101, were incapable of causing cholera gravis. They were highly immunogenic and showed protection following administration of a single oral dose. However, they exhibited unacceptable residual reactogenicity. CVD 103, derived from a classical Inaba wild-type parent, was the first live oral cholera vaccine strain to be well tolerated and highly immunogenic and protective following ingestion of a single oral dose. The current single-dose live oral cholera strain CVD103-HgR, which is a licensed vaccine in many countries, is a further derivative of CVD 103.

In 1978, CVD investigators settled an important controversy that raged over whether so-called enteropathogenic *E. coli* (EPEC) of classical infantile diarrhea O.H Serotypes were inherently able to cause diarrhea, even though they did not elaborate LT or ST enterotoxins and did not exhibit *Shigella*-like invasiveness. The ability of several such strains to cause overt diarrhea was irrefutably demonstrated in a volunteer challenge study. Once this observation was made, CVD investigators began to search for virulence factors responsible for causing the diarrhea. Dr. Kaper launched this research into a new level of sophistication by application of bacterial genetic techniques. This approach began with the demonstration that EPEC carry a circa 60 MD plasmid involved in attaching to epithelial cells.

In the early 1980s, Jim Kaper succeeded in competing for two separate RO1 grants. For the next two decades, he successfully held at least two separate concomitantly running RO1 grants, and grants-in-aid from other funding sources.

Two other colleagues who played key roles during this period were Dr. Mary Lou Clements, who served as Chief of the Adult Clinical Studies Section from 1979 to 1985 and Dr. Robert E. Black, who was Chief of the Epidemiology Section of the CVD from 1980 to 1985.

1984–1997: THE CVD, THE DIVISION OF GEOGRAPHIC MEDICINE, AND THE DIVISION OF INFECTIOUS DISEASES AND TROPICAL PEDIATRICS

In 1984, the Division of Infectious Diseases of the Department of Medicine, including the CVD, moved to the Medical School Teaching Facility (MSTF) at South Pine Street, which had notably improved laboratory facilities and office space. The years 1984 and 1985 were hallmark years in the evolution of the CVD. In 1984, Dr. John Kastor assumed the chairmanship of the Department of Medicine; acting on the recommendations of Drs. Theodore E. Woodward and Stephen C. Schimpff (Director of the Division), Dr. Kastor and the medical school administration made the CVD a separate division within the Department of Medicine, the Division of Geographic Medicine. The Division of Geographic Medicine CVD continued to work closely with the Division of Infectious Diseases, and the two divisions sponsored a joint fellowship program for internists pursuing infectious diseases training. Beginning in 1984, other major changes occurred that led to a fundamental alteration both in structure and in the modus operandi of the CVD. In 1984, I was appointed Acting Head of the Division of Infectious Diseases of the Department of Pediatrics and in 1985 accepted this full-time post with the provision that the name be changed to the Division of Infectious Diseases and Tropical Pediatrics. This more closely reflected the direction in which we hoped to lead that division with an interest in the infectious diseases of children in developing countries. All faculty members of the Division of Infectious Diseases and Tropical Pediatrics were expected to be fully integrated members of the CVD and to carry out research in a discipline of vaccinology. Hence, in 1985, the CVD truly became a center that crossed departmental lines. In 1992, with the arrival of Dr. Alessio Fasano as the Head of the Division of Gastroenterology and Nutrition in the Department of Pediatrics, the faculty of this third division joined the CVD. In 1995, the CVD moved to new quarters in the Medical School Teaching Facility, having been assigned excellent facilities on the third and fourth floors.

In the 1990s, the CVD constitutes a multidisciplinary entity with a total staff of approximately 85 professionals, including approximately 26 full-time faculty. Another 45 staff members work in the center's field unit, "CVD-Chile," in Santiago, Chile. A new field unit was established in Mali, West Africa in 1997. Year after year during this period, CVD investigators recruited 6 to 8 million dollars in competitive grants and contracts for support of research activities; most of these grants were from the NIH. These included many RO1s, NO1s, and UO1s. Research activities of the CVD cover many aspects of vaccinology, including basic research (e.g., pathogenesis, construction of vaccine candidates and fundamental immunologic studies), clinical vaccine evaluation (Phase 1 and 2 clinical trials of many vaccines in adult and pediatric subjects), sophisticated measurements of immune responses and field epidemiologic studies (e.g., Phase 3 efficacy trials, post-licensure effectiveness trials, and serosurveys). Many faculty members have made major contributions to the growth and maintenance of the CVD in the 1980s and 1990s, almost too numerous to record. Nevertheless, the contributions of Margaret Rennels, Deirdre Herrington, Carol Tacket, Genevieve Losonsky, Robert Edelman, Steven Wasserman, J. Glenn Morris, Karen Kotloff, James Nataro, Rosanna Lagos, John Clemens, Bradford Kay, and Caterine Ferreccio merit special mention.

The CVD fulfills a vigorous and varied teaching program on several levels. The CVD trains internists (through the combined fellowship program with the Division of Infectious Diseases in the Department of Medicine), pediatricians (through the pediatric infectious disease fellowship), and Ph.D. postdoctoral fellows. Doctoral students from the Department of Microbiology and Immunology eagerly pursue their research thesis projects through mentor sponsorship in the CVD. In 1997, the CVD was awarded the first-ever NIH training grant in vaccinology, a prestigious T32 grant that will be active for five years. In the extraordinary year of 1997, the CVD was signally awarded a second

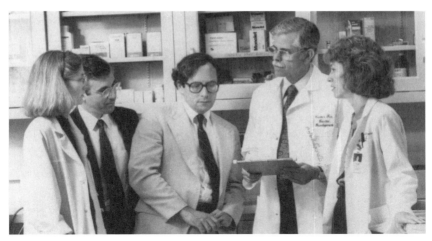

Left to right: Carol O. Tacket, M.D., Steven S. Wasserman, Ph.D., John D. Clemens, M.D., Robert Edelman, M.D., Deirdre A. Herrington, M.D.

five-year training grant in emerging infections as part of a national competition NIH sponsorship of the Fogarty Institute of NIH.

Single-dose live oral cholera vaccine strain CVD 103-HgR became a licensed vaccine in 1994 in Switzerland. During the next two years, many other countries, including Canada, licensed CVD 103-HgR. A series of other live oral vaccines are under development by CVD investigators, including attenuated *Salmo-*

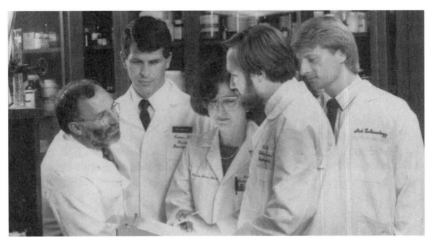

Left to right: Myron M. Levine, M.D., D.T.P.H., Bradford A. Kay, MS, Dr. P.H. Suzanne Giannini, Ph.D., James B. Kaper, M.D., Jonathan R. Davis, Ph.D.

nella typhi and *Shigella* strains. They are in various stages of clinical trials.

The CVD has come a long way from its humble beginnings. At present, the CVD constitutes the largest academic vaccinology research unit in the world. Over the years, the CVD has contributed significantly to enhance the long tradition of excellence for the study and practice of infectious diseases at the University of Maryland School of Medicine.

Margaret (Peggy) B. Rennels, M.D., Professor of Pediatrics and a 1973 medical school graduate, has contributed importantly to the control of diarrheal disorders, particularly rotavirus infections in children. Her fundamental studies conducted in Baltimore and throughout Maryland have shown convincingly that rotavirus vaccines, given orally, prevent illness and markedly reduce morbidity, mortality and the need for hospitalization and patient-doctor visits. The incidence of intussusception has limited its use. Dr. Rennels has performed her research collaboratively with the infectious diseases divisions of the Department of Pediatrics, Medicine and the Center for Vaccine Development. She

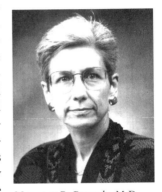

Margaret B. Rennels, M.D.
Professor of Pediatrics

is a superb teacher and a recognized authority in epidemiology and preventive medicine. Her other studies and research interests have embraced pneumococcal and meningococcal vaccines.

REFERENCES

1. Black RE, Cisneros L, Levine MM, Banfi A, Lobos H, Rodriguez H. A case-control study to identify risk factors for endemic typhoid fever in Santiago, Chile. Bull. World Health Org. 1985;63:899–904.

2. Herrington DA, Clyde DF, Losonsky GL, Cortesia M, Murphy JR, David J, Baqar S, Felix AM, Heiner EP, Gillesen D, Nardin EH, Nussenzweig RS, Nussenzweig V, Hollingdale MR, Levine MM. Safety and immunogenicity in man of a synthetic peptide malaria vaccine against *Plasmodium falciparum* sporozoites. Nature 1987;328:257–259.

3. Levine MM, Ferreccio C, Black RE, Chilean Typhoid Committee, Germanier R. Large-scale field trial of Ty21a live oral typhoid vaccine in enteric-coated capsule formulation. Lancet 1987;8541:1049–1052.

4. Levine MM, Kaper JB, Herrington D, Ketley J, Losonsky G, Tacket CO, Tall B, Cryz S. Safety, immunogenicity, and efficacy of recombinant live oral cholera vaccines, CVD 103 and CVD 103-HgR. Lancet 1988;ii:467–470.

5. Tacket CO, Losonsky G, Link H, Hoang Y, Guesry P, Hilpert H, Levine MM. Protective efficacy of a milk immunoglobulin concentrate against oral challenge with enterotoxigenic *Escherichia coli*. New England J. Med. 1988;318:1240–1243.

6. Jerse AE, Yu J, Tall BD, Kaper JB. A genetic locus of enteropathogenic *Escherichia coli* necessary for production of attaching and effacing lesions on tissue culture cells. Proc. Nat. Acad. Sci., USA 1990;87: 7839–7843.

7. Ferreccio C, Prado V, Ojeda A, Cayazzo M, Abrego P, Guers L, Levine MM. Epidemiologic patterns of acute diarrhea and endemic *Shigella* infections in a poor periurban setting in Santiago, Chile. Amer. J. Epidemiol. 1991;134:614–627.

8. Fasano A, Baudry-Maurelli B, Pumplin DW, Wasserman SS, Tall BD, Ketley JM, Kaper JB. *Vibrio cholerae* produces a second enterotoxin which affects intestinal tight junctions. Proc. Nat. Acad. Sci, USA 1991; 88:5242–5246.

9. Sztein MB, Tanner MK, Polotsky Y, Orenstein JM, Levine MM. Cytotoxic lymphocytes after oral immunization with attenuated strains of *Salmonella typhi* in humans. J. Immunol. 1995;155:3987–3993.

10. Lagos R, Horwitz I, Toro J, San Martin O, Abrego P, Bustamante C, Wasserman SS, Levine OS, Levine MM. Large scale postlicensure, selective vaccination of Chilean infants with PRP-T conjugate vaccine: practicality and effectiveness in preventing invasive *Haemophilus influenzae* type b infections. Pediatr Infect. Dis. J. 1996;15:216–222.

11. Karaolis DK, Johnson JA, Bailey CC, Boedeker EC, Kaper JB, Reeves PR. A *Vibrio cholerae* pathogenicity island associated with epidemic and pandemic strains. Proc. Natl. Acad. Sci. U.S.A. 1998;95:3134–9.

12. Tacket CO, Mason HS, Losonsky G, Clements JD, Levine MM, Arntzen CJ. Immunogenicity in humans of a recombinant bacterial antigen delivered in a transgenic potato. Nature Medicine 1998;4:607–609.

ADDITIONAL REFERENCES

Rennels MB, Glass RI, Dennehy PH, Bernstein DI, Pichichero ME, Zito ET, Mack ME, Davidson BL, Zapikian AZ. Safety and efficacy of high-dose Rhesus-human reassortant rotavirus vaccines—report of the National Multicenter Trial. Ped 1996;97:7–13.

Rennels MB, Edwards KM, Keyserling HL, Reisinger KS, Hogerman DA, Chang I, Paradiso PR, Malinoski FJ, Kumura A. Safety and immunogenicity of heptavalent pneumococcal vaccine conjugated to CRM$_{197}$ in United States infants. Ped 1998;101:604–611.

Nalin DR, Cash RA, Islan R, Motta M, Phillips RA. Oral maintenance therapy for cholera in adults. Lancet 1968;2370.

Hornick RB, DuPont HL, Levine MM, Gilman RH, Woodward WE, Snyder MJ, and Woodward TE. Efficacy of a live oral typhoid vaccine in human volunteers. Div. Biol. Standards 1995;33: 89–92.

Gilman RH, Hornick RB, Woodward WE, DuPont HL, Snyder MJ, Levine MM, Libonati JP. Evaluation of a UDP Glocose-4 epimetaseless mutant of salmonella typhi as a live oral vaccine. J Infect Dis 1977;136:717–723.

Tacket CO, Hone DM, Losonsky GA, Guera L, Edelman R, Levine MM. Clinical acceptability and immunogenicity of CVD 908 salmonella typhi vaccine strain. Vaccine 1992;10(7):443–446.

Woodward WE, Gilman RH, Hornick RB, Libonati JP, Cash RA. Efficacy of a live oral cholera vaccine in human volunteers. Fourteenth Congress of the International Association of Biological Standardization. Douglas, Isle of Man, 1975. Develop Biol Standard 33:108–112 (S. Karget, Basel 1976).

Levine MM, Kaper JB, Herrington D, Ketley J, Losonsky G, Tacket CO, Tall B. Safety, immunogenicity, and efficacy of Cryz, S recombinant live oral cholera vaccines, CVD 103, and CVD 108-HgR. Lancet 1988;27(August):467–470.

20

DIVISION OF INFECTIOUS DISEASES, 1985–1996

John W. Warren, M.D.

In October 1985, Stephen C. Schimpff, M.D., resigned as both the Head of the Division of Infectious Diseases and as the Director of the University of Maryland Cancer Center to become the Executive Vice President of the University of Maryland Medical Systems. I was named Acting Head and became permanent Head in August 1986. I had received my medical degree and training in infectious diseases at Harvard Medical School.

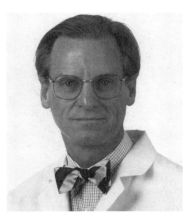

John W. Warren, M.D.

The Division experienced a great deal of growth in the 10 years since 1986. Over this period of time, the Division grew from 6 to 21 faculty members, the latter group composed of 18 M.D.s and three Ph.D.s. This growth can best be described in three important Division activities: research, clinical work, and teaching.

RESEARCH

In 1986, the Division's research was in two main areas: antibiotic studies funded mostly by pharmaceutical companies and work on catheter-associated urinary tract infections (UTI) funded by the National Institutes of Health. Over the next 10 years, basic research in the Division was greatly strengthened in three areas.

Molecular Bacterial Pathogenesis

The first area involved the use of the powerful tools of molecular and cellular biology to study interactions of bacterial strains and human epithelial cells, a discipline described as molecular bacterial pathogenesis. In general, the scheme used by these investigators was to observe a bacteria–epithelial cell interaction, develop assays to measure this interaction, and then determine probable mechanisms of pathogenesis by manipulating the bacterial genome or the epithelial cell response.

Building upon our clinical and epidemiologic studies, we exploited the revolution in molecular biology to develop research in the molecular pathogenesis of urinary tract infection (UTI).[1–9] While much was known of properties of pyelonephritogenic *Escherichia coli*, little was understood of the means by which these organisms interacted with the host to cause disease. Four faculty members were recruited who have helped to develop these concepts.

Harry L.T. Mobley, Ph.D., obtained his Ph.D. at the University of Louisville School of Medicine and acquired postdoctoral training with James Kaper, Ph.D., at the University of Maryland. Dr. Mobley initiated a series of investigations into the molecular pathogeneses of UTIs caused by *E. coli* and *Proteus mirabilis*. In regard to the former, he developed isogenic mutants (e.g., P fimbriae and hemolysin) to test in animal models and in human renal epithelial cell cultures. For *P. mirabilis*, he identified numerous virulence factors and discovered a new fimbriae, becoming probably the foremost

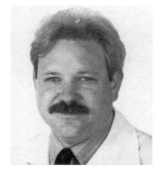

Harry L.T. Mobley, Ph.D.

expert on *P. mirabilis* infections. Additionally, based on his work with urease in *P. mirabilis*, he became intrigued with this enzyme in *Helicobacter pylori*, the agent of gastritis and gastric and duodenal ulcer. Here too he has become renowned for his ability to decipher the virulence of this gastric pathogen.[3–7,9–11]

Michael S. Donnenberg, M.D., was recruited to the University of Maryland by way of Columbia and Tufts. At the latter institution during his fellowship in infectious diseases, he became

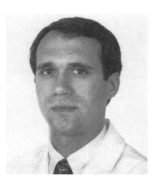

Michael S. Donnenberg, M.D.

intrigued by the mechanisms of pathogenesis of enteropathogenic *E. coli*. By using transposon mutagenesis, Dr. Donnenberg demonstrated several steps in the pathogenesis of this organism and at Maryland undertook molecular biologic means to understand the mechanisms of infection. Thereby, he opened an entire field of inquiry now being pursued by numerous investigators across the world. He applied similar techniques to studies of interaction of uropathogenic *E. coli* and renal epithelial cells.[6,12–18]

Michael D. Island, Ph.D., obtained his Ph.D. at the University of Tennessee and became a postdoctoral fellow in the Division and subsequently a faculty member

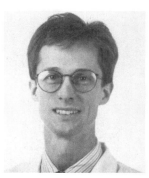

Michael D. Island, Ph.D.

in 1995. His interest was in the relatively unexplored area of pathogenesis of bacterial cystitis, a very common infection, but one whose pathogenesis is little understood. His work in *E. coli* was devoted to understanding adherence, cytotoxicity, and the role of cytotoxic necrotizing factor and their effects upon bladder epithelial cells.

Supporting this work in UTIs was David E. Johnson, Ph.D., who adapted a mouse model of urinary tract infection which he and others have shown to be useful in distinguishing bacterial strains causing pyelonephritis from those causing cystitis from fecal isolates of the same species. This model is similarly useful for distinguishing bacterial strains isogenic but for the

presence or absence of a putative virulence factor.[3–5,9,19]

Additionally, the Division expanded
its molecular pathogenesis work to include enteric organisms. J. Glenn Morris,
M.D., M.P.H., T.M., received his training at Tulane, University of Texas Southwestern, Emory, and the CDC before un-
dertaking a fellowship in Infectious
Diseases at the University of Maryland.
He became highly recognized as an expert on enteric toxins and *Vibrio* surface

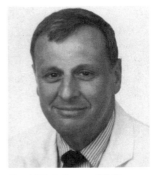

David E. Johnson, Ph.D.

polysaccharides and has studied *V. vulnificus* and the non-Ol *V.
cholerae* including *V. cholerae* 0139 Bengal.[19] His work on enteric pathogens was of such a caliber that he was asked to take a
partial sabbatical in 1995 and 1996 at the U.S. Department of
Agriculture to reconstruct microbiologic methods for food safety,
a program that had not been changed since the early 1900s.

Acute Inflammation

The second area of research expertise within the Division and
one complementing that in bacterial pathogenesis comprised
three faculty members interested in the acute inflammatory response. Simeon E. Goldblum, M.D., by way of Einstein, New
Mexico, and Kentucky, studied features of infectious agents and
the host response that compromise pulmonary vascular endothelial barrier function, demonstrating that certain bacterial components and endogenous mediators can induce capillary leaks. He
demonstrated a structure–function rela-
tionship between actin reorganization
and changes in barrier function, and
began to unravel the mechanisms of
these changes. These findings are of importance in adult respiratory distress
syndrome and other diseases in which
capillary leakage is part of the pathogenesis.[20–24]

Alan S. Cross, M.D., was recruited
after a career at Walter Reed Army Institute of Research to come to the Univer-

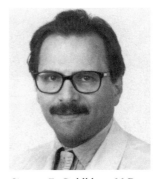

Simeon E. Goldblum, M.D.

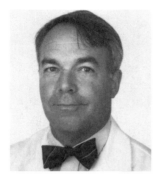

Alan S. Cross, M.D.

sity of Maryland in 1994. His work embraced systemic Gram-negative bacterial infections and immunologic strategies against these infections. His work in basic mechanisms of endotoxin and cytokine physiology gained him national prominence, and his work in Baltimore was dedicated to understanding the beneficial and detrimental roles that host signals induced by endotoxin play in normal host defenses.

Michael E. Kleinberg, M.D., Ph.D., who trained at Einstein, Cornell, and the NIH, studied mechanisms by which the superoxide-producing NADPH oxidase complex of myeloid phagocytes is activated from its dormant state. His work led him into molecular and cell biology and the pathogenesis of acute inflammation. His work will have important implications beyond understanding the respiratory burst when similar proteins are found in a large number of signal transduction pathways.[25–27]

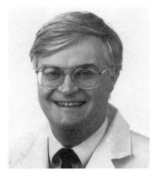

Michael E. Kleinberg, M.D., Ph.D.

Virology

More recently, a group of young investigators interested in basic virologic research were recruited to the Division. These include

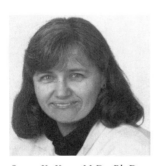

Susan K. Keay, M.D., Ph.D.

Susan Keay, M.D., Ph.D., who came from a fellowship at Stanford and whose interest in the cell receptor for cytomegalovirus led her to an understanding of cell biology and signal transduction induced by this virus.[8,27–30] Priscilla Furth, M.D., by way of Yale and Harvard, joined the Division as a clinician. She took a three-year sabbatical leave to learn virology and returned as a skilled virologist for work in viral oncogenesis, the role of apoptosis in breast cancer, and gene transfer into somatic tissue.[31-35] David Oldach, M.D., who received his medical degree at the University of Maryland and served his residency at Massachusetts General Hospital and his fellowship at Johns Hopkins, returned as a Maryland faculty member. Through his clinical work in the transplant program, he became interested in hepatitis C virus and developed in vitro and in vivo models to study this infection.[30] David M. Margolis, M.D., after training at Tufts, the NIH, and University of Massachusetts, came to the University of Maryland to study HIV and gene therapy.

Although there are many measures of research productivity, one involves the amount and source of funding. In 1986, the Division's research budget totaled $758,000, much of it in a program project grant on urinary tract infections. By 1996, Division investigators were receiving almost $4 million in annual grants, almost $3 million of this derived from the NIH and other federal agencies.

CLINICAL WORK

The Division's clinical activities also grew substantially and by 1996 comprised four busy services. The most venerable was the University/VA service, which supervised general community and nosocomial infections in these two hospitals; this service averaged about 60 patients per month. Additionally, by 1996, there were three subspecialty services, each with a director and a small cadre of faculty who are experts in these areas. These included the solid organ transplant ID program, which served the renal, pancreas, liver, heart, and lung transplantation services; this program grew rapidly after 1992 and by 1996 involved approximately 90 inpatient consultations per month. The Cancer Center ID program consulted for about 35 patients per month, mostly those with leukemia, lymphoma, or bone marrow transplants. The third service was the HIV Program. This comprised an HIV ward structured as one of the Department of Medicine rotations. It was implemented by an ID attending and fellow, as well as by residents and medical students. Additionally, the HIV program sponsored several clinics, each with an HIV-dedicated attending physician as well as fellows and other health care providers.

The 18 physicians in the Division and three in the Division of Geographic Medicine comprised the Division's 21 attending doctors for its clinical services in 1996. In toto, the Division, by 1996, cared for upwards of 250 inpatients per month and about 300 outpatients per month. The income from clinical services for FY 96 approximated $900,000, compared to the clinical income for FY 1986 of about $90,000.

EDUCATION

With the introduction of problem-based learning to the medical curriculum, the Division faculty by 1996 took increasing academic responsibility, particularly in teaching microbiology and infectious diseases to second-year medical students. Its molecular biologists conducted an important course in this subject to the medical school's graduate students. Teaching of residents, third- and fourth-year medical students occurred primarily on the HIV ward and the University/VA consulting service.

The Fellowship program attracted about 35 applicants in 1985. By 1996 about 90 candidates applied per year. Usually the Fellowship program attracted three to four new fellows, for a two-year clinical track or a three-year (or more) research track. For fellows, the Division developed a didactic course of weekly lectures which, over a two-year period, present a complete review of the field of infectious diseases. Additionally, a monthly journal club is conducted for fellows and faculty participation. Finally, the Division sponsors an annual visiting professor program. Three to five recognized authorities of various infectious diseases spend two days with faculty members and fellows for discussion of problems of mutual interest.

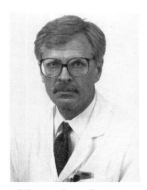

Dr. Philip A. Mackowiak was recruited from Dallas in 1988 to head the medical service at the Baltimore Veterans Administration Medical Center. Immediately, he became very active in the educational program for medical students and house officers, which included performing attending and consultative responsibilities for the Infectious Diseases Division. His

Philip Mackowiak, M.D.

particular authoritative forte is fever. His scholarly work performed in congenial collaboration with others culminated in two comprehensive monographs on fever in 1991 and 1997. The initial significance of pyrexia, its characterization, mediators, pathogenesis, methods of detection and management.

INSTITUTE OF HUMAN VIROLOGY

In the mid-1990s, the Division entered a new phase of growth. This was initiated by the recruitment of Edmund Tramont, M.D., who after a long successful career in infectious diseases in the Army Medical Corps was recruited to head the Medical Biotechnology Center of the University of Maryland Biotechnology Institute.

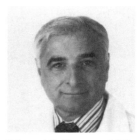

Dr. Tramont subsequently recruited Robert C. Gallo, M.D., Robert R. Redfield, M.D., and William A. Blattner, M.D., to form the Institute of Human Virology in the Medical Biotechnology Center. This group arrived in 1995 with plans to develop an extremely strong team devoted to basic epidemiologic and clinical research in viral diseases. The emphasis involves not only HIV infection but other

Edmund C. Tramont, M.D.

chronic viruses and characterization of newly recognized human viral pathogens.

All members of the Institute have joint appointments with medical school groups. Dr. Redfield's appointment is with the Division of Infectious Diseases. Building upon a solid base of good clinical care, a program constructed by Harold Standiford, M.D.,

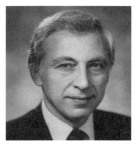
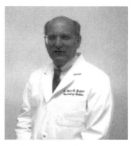
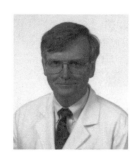

Robert C. Gallo, M.D.   *Robert R. Redfield, M.D.*   *William A. Blattner, M.D.*

David Wheeler, M.D., Jonathan Cohn, M.D., M.P.H., and Claire Beiser, M.D., M.P.H., Dr. Redfield is charged with developing a large, dynamic, multidisciplinary HIV clinical research program. The Division and Institute have established a close relationship and will build upon it a cadre of competent investigators, stressing joint appointments and collaborators.

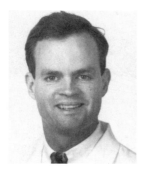 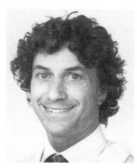 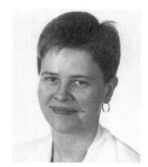

David A. Wheeler, M.D.   *Jonathan A. Cohn, M.D., M.P.H.*   *Claire L. Beiser, M.D., M.P.H.*

THE FUTURE

The Division intends to maintain its prominence in the molecular pathogenesis of bacterial infections and to enhance its research of acute inflammatory disorders. However, the most prominent growth likely will be in basic and clinical virologic research, particularly HIV, conducted in close collaboration with the Institute of Human Virology. With relation to clinical problems, the Division is positioning itself to meet the challenges offered by the oncoming era of managed care and foresees growth in its solid organ transplant and HIV/AIDS programs and, to a lesser extent, in its program for cancer and bone marrow transplant patients.

REFERENCES

1. Warren JW, Damron D, Tenney JH, Hoopes JM, Deforge B, Muncie Jr HL. Fever, bacteremia, and death as complications of bacteriuria in women with long-term urethral catheters. J Infect Dis 1987;155:1151–1158.

2. Warren JW, Muncie Jr HL, Hall-Craggs M. Acute pyelonephritis associated with the bacteriuria of long-term catheterizations: a prospective clinicopathological study. J Infect Dis 1988;158:1341-1346.

3. Jones BD, Lockatell CV, Johnson DE, Warren JW, Mobley HLT. Construction of a urease negative mutant of *Proteus mirabilis*: Analysis of virulence in a mouse model of ascending urinary tract infection. Infect Immun 1990;58:1120–1123.

4. Johnson DE, Russell RG, Lockatell CV, Mobley HLT, Warren JW. Contribution of *Proteus mirabilis* urease to persistence, urolithiasis, and renal pathology in a mouse model of ascending urinary tract infection. Infect Immun 1993;61:2748–2754.

5. Bahrani FK, Massad G, Lockatell CV, Johnson DE, Russell RG, Warren JW, Mobley HLT. Construction of an MR/P fimbrial mutant of *Proteus mirabilis:* Role in virulence in a mouse model of ascending urinary tract infection. Infect Immun 1994;62:3363–3371.

6. Trifillis AL, Donnenberg MS, Cui X, Russell RG, Utsalo SJ, Mobley HLT, Warren JW. Binding to and killing of human renal epithelial cells by hemolytic P-fimbriated *Escherichia coli*. Kidney Int 1994;46:1083–1091.

7. Mobley HLT, Warren JW. Urinary tract infections: Molecular pathogenesis and clinical management. American Society for Microbiology: Washington, D.C., 1996.

8. Keay S, Zhang C-O, Hise M, Trifillis AL, Hebel JR, Jacobs SC, Warren JW. Decreased ^{3}H-thymidine incorporation by human bladder epithelial cells following exposure to urine from interstitial cystitis patients. J Urol 1996;156:2073–2078.

9. Mobley HLT, Belas R, Lockatell V, Chippendale G, Trifillis AL, Johnson DE, Warren JW. Construction of a flagellum-negative mutant of *Proteus mirabilis*: Effect on internalization by human renal epithelial cells and virulence in a mouse model of ascending urinary tract infection. Infect Immun 1996;64:5332–5340.

10. Jones BD, Mobley HLT. *Proteus mirabilis* urease: Genetic organization, regulation, and expression of structural genes. J Bacteriol 1988;170:3342–3349.

11. Mobley HLT, Cortesia MJ, Jones BD. Characterization of urease from *Campylobacter pylori*. J Clin Microbiol 1988;26:831–836.

12. Donnenberg MS, Tacket CO, James SP, Losonsky G, Nataro JP, Wasserman SS, Kaper JB, Levine MM. The role of the *eaeA* gene in experimental enteropathogenic *Escherichia coli* infection. J Clin Invest 1993;92:1412–1417.

13. Donnenberg MS, Tzipori S, McKee ML, O'Brien AD, Alroy J, Kaper JB. The role of the *eae* gene of enterohemorrhagic *Escherichia coli* in intimate attachment *in vitro* and in a porcine model. J Clin Invest 1993;92:1418–1424.

14. Kenny B, Lai L-C, Finlay BB, Donnenberg MS. EspA, a protein secreted by enteropathogenic *Escherichia coli*, is required to induce signals in epithelial cells. Molec Microbiol 1996;20:313–323.

15. Rabinowitz RP, Lai L-C, Jarvis K, McDaniel TK, Kaper JB, Stone KD, Donnenberg MS. Attaching and effacing of host cells by enteropathogenic *Escherichia coli* in the absence of detectable tyrosine kinase mediated signal transduction. Microb Pathogen 96;21:157–171.

16. Stone KD, Zhang H-Z, Carlson LK, Donnenberg MS. A cluster of fourteen genes from enteropathogenic *Escherichia coli* is sufficient for biogenesis of a type IV pilus. Molec Microbiol 1996;20:325–337.

17. Lai L-C, Wainwright LA, Stone KD, Donnenberg MS. A third secreted protein that is encoded by the enteropathogenic *Escherichia coli* pathogenicity island is required for transduction of signals and for attaching and effacing activities in host cells. Infect Immun 1997;65: 2211–2217.

18. Donnenberg MS, Zhang H-Z, Stone KD. Biogenesis of the bundle-forming pilus of enteropathogenic *Escherichia coli*: Reconstitution of fimbriae in recombinant *E. coli* and role of DsbA in pilin stability. Gene 1997;192:33–38.

19. Morris JG, Wright AC, Simpson LM, Wood RK, Johnson DE, Oliver JD. Virulence of *Vibrio vulnificus*: Association with utilization of transferrin-bound iron, and lack of correlation with levels of protease production. FEMS Microbiol Letters 1987;40:55–59.

20. Goldblum SE, Sun WL. Human recombinant tumor necrosis factor augments pulmonary artery transendothelial albumin flux *in vitro*. Am J Physiol 1990;258:L57–L67.

21. Goldblum SE, Ding X, Brann TW, Campbell-Washington J. Bacterial lipopolysaccharide induces actin reorganization, intercellular gap formation and endothelial barrier dysfunction in pulmonary vascular endothelial cells. Concurrent F-actin depolymerization and new actin synthesis. J Cell Physiol 1993;157:13–23.

22. Goldblum SE, Brann TW, Ding X, Pugin J, Tobias PS. Lipopolysaccharide (LPS)-binding protein (LBP) and soluble CD14 function as accessory molecules for LPS-induced changes in endothelial barrier function. J Clin Invest 1994;93:692–702.

23. Goldblum SE, Ding X, Funk S, Sage EH. SPARC regulates cell shape and endothelial barrier function. Proc Natl Acad Sci USA 1994; 91:3448–3452.

24. Bannerman DD, Goldblum SE. Endotoxin induces endothelial barrier dysfunction through protein tyrosine phosphorylation. Am J Physiol 1997;273:L217–L226.

25. Kleinberg ME, Malech HL, Rotrosen D. The phagocyte 47 kilo-dalton cytosolic oxidase protein is an early reactant in activation of the respiratory burst. J Biol Chem 1990;265:15577–15583.

26. Kleinberg ME, Malech HL, Mital D, Leto TL. P47-*phox* is the first cytosol protein to participate in formation of the phagocyte NADPH oxidase. Biochemistry 1994;22:2490–2495.

27. Baldwin BR, Kleinberg M, Keay S. Molecular cloning and expression of receptor peptides that block human cytomegalovirus/cell fusion. Biochem Biophys Res Commun 1996;219:668–673.

28. Keay S, Baldwin B. Anti-idiotype antibodies that mimic gp 86 of human cytomegalovirus inhibit viral fusion but not attachment. J Virol 1991;65:5124–5128.

29. Keay S, Baldwin B. The human fibroblast receptor for gp86 of human cytomegalovirus is a phosphorylated glycoprotein. J Virol 1992; 66:4834-4838.

30. Keay S, Oldach DW, Wiland SA, Klassen D, Schweitzer E, Bartlett B, Abruzzo L, Kuman D. Post-transplant lymphoproliferative disorder associated with OKT3 and decreased antiviral prophylaxis in pancreas transplant recipients. Clin Infect Dis 1997.

31. Furth PA. Heterosexual transmission of AIDS by male drug abusers. Nature 1987;327:193.

32. Furth PA, Kerr D, Wall R. Gene transfer by jet injection into differentiated tissues of living animals and in organ culture. Mol Biotechnol 1995;4:121–127.

33. Furth PA, St. Onge L, Boger H, Gruss P, Gossen M, Kisner A, Bujard H, Hennighausen L. Temporal control of gene expression in transgenic mice by a tetracycline responsive promoter in transgenic mice. Proc Natl Acad Sci USA 1994;91:9302–9306.

34. Ewald D, Li M, Efrat S, Wall RJ, Furth PA, Hennighausen L. Time-sensitive reversal of hyperplasia in transgenic mice expressing SV40T antigen. Science 1996;273:1384–1386.

35. Li M, Liu X, Robinson T, Bar-Peled U, Wagner K-U, Young WS, Hennighausen L, Furth PA. Mammary derived signals activate programmed cell death during the first stage of mammary gland involution. Proc Natl Acad Sci USA 1997;94:3425–3430.

ADDITIONAL REFERENCES

Bilello JA, Eiseman JL, Standiford HC, Drusano GL. Impact of dosing schedule upon suppression of a retrovirus in a murine model of AIDS encephalopathy. Antimicrob Agents Chemother 1994;38: 628–631.

Drusano GL, Plaisance KI, Forrest A, Standiford HC. Dose ranging study and constant infusion evaluation of ciprofloxacin. Antimicrob Agents Chemother 1986;30:444–446.

Khabbaz RF, Kaper JB, Moody MR, Schimpff SC, Tenney JH. Molecular epidemiology of group JK *Corynebacterium*: Lack of evidence for patient to patient transmission. J Infect Dis 1986;154:95–99.

Perlman D, Caplan ES. Nosocomial sinusitis: a new and complex threat. J Crit Illness 1987;2(5):19–25.

Tenney JH, Moody MR, Newman KA, Schimpff SC, Wade JC, Coster-ton JW, Reed WP. Adherent microorganisms on lumenal surfaces of long-term intravenous catheters: Importance of *S. epidermidis* in cancer patients. Arch Intern Med 1986;146:1949–1955.

21

ACTIVITIES OF THE INSTITUTE OF HUMAN VIROLOGY

Jennifer Schorr in collaboration
with Robert C. Gallo, M.D.

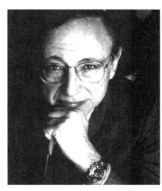

Robert C. Gallo, M.D.

In 1995, Robert C. Gallo, M.D., of the National Cancer Institute, Robert R. Redfield, M.D., of the Walter Reed Army Medical Center, and William A. Blattner, M.D., of the National Cancer Institute were recruited by Edmund Tramont, M.D., to form the Institute of Human Virology (IHV). The IHV is a center in the University of Maryland Biotechnology Institute and is located at the Medical Biotechnology Center on the University of Maryland, Baltimore Campus. Formally inaugurated in November of 1996, the IHV is comprised of an extremely strong and synergistic professional team devoted to research on viral diseases and virally linked cancers. The IHV at the University of Maryland was established to create and develop a world-class center of excellence focusing on chronic viral diseases and virally linked cancers. The IHV is dedicated to discovery, re-

227

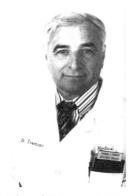

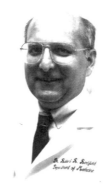

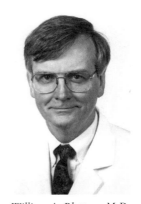

Edmund C. Tramont, M.D.
Professor of Medicine

Robert A. Redfield, M.D.
Professor of Medicine

William A. Blattner, M.D.
Professor of Medicine

search, treatment, and prevention of these diseases and cancers. Its unique structure seeks to connect cohesive, multidisciplinary research and clinical programs so that new treatments are streamlined from discovery to patient. The IHV serves patients locally and the scientific community globally. Its five principal, interrelated divisions are: Basic Science, Epidemiology and Prevention, Vaccine Development, Clinical Care and Research, and Animal Models. Over half of the faculty have joint appointments with departments in the Medical or Pharmacy Schools. Dr. Gallo is the Director of the Institute and Professor of Medicine at the University of Maryland, Baltimore.

CHEMOKINE RESEARCH

The study of chemokines is the principal research interest of Dr. Gallo, co-discoverer of HIV-1, and a team of researchers he recruited to the Institute, including Fiorenza Cocchi, M.D., Anthony DeVico, Ph.D., and Alfredo Garzino-Demo, Ph.D.[1] They identified several chemokines that suppress HIV-1 infection by blocking the chemokine receptors required by HIV-1 to gain entry into cells. While collaborating with other investigators in France and Italy, Gallo showed that excess production of chemokines was most likely responsible for the ability of hemophiliacs (repeatedly exposed intravenously to HIV-1) to remain uninfected by the virus. HIV researchers continue to study chemokines and their receptors, aimed at elucidating the mechanisms by which these substances prevent or suppress HIV infection. The work will help determine whether the suppressive properties of chemokines can be exploited to produce effective drugs and biological vaccines for HIV-1 infection (AIDS).

CONTROL OF CANCER

Another highly regarded area of research at the IHV is under direction of Gallo, Joseph Bryant, D.V.M., and Yanto Lunardi-Isklandar on compounds known as hCG-associated factors (HAF).[2] While studying Kaposi's sarcoma (KS), the researchers and investigators at the University of Brussels and the University of Southern California showed that HAF inhibited HIV replication in vitro, blocked infection in monkeys infected with Simian Immunodeficiency Virus (SIV), and diminshed KS tumors in approximately half of the patients treated with the compound. Some treated patients experienced improved energy levels, weight gain, and boosted CD4 cell counts. The anti-tumor activity of HAF does not appear to be limited to KS, but applies to other cancers as well. These researchers are now purifying and identifying the molecular components and structure of HAF. The ultimate objective is to generate large quantities for practical use.

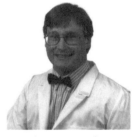

David M. Hone, Ph.D.

The IHV's Division of Vaccine Research focuses on developing innovative vaccines for delivery systems against a variety of chronic viral diseases. David Hone, Ph.D., and George Lewis, Ph.D., developed an oral HIV-1 mucosal vaccine using an avirulent *Salmonella* strain as a vaccine vector.[3,4] Unlike most HIV vaccines, which are designed to activate B cells, the Hone–Lewis vaccine activates T cells. Such activity correlates with protection from HIV infection in animal models. The vaccine is being tested in clinical trials.

Hone and Lewis developed a patented method for use of bacteria to deliver genes expressed by the animal cells the bacteria infects rather that by the bacteria themselves. This "batoinfection" technique enables creation of vaccines that are less expensive and time-consuming to produce than DNA vaccines or those created by using viruses as vectors. This will be useful in the development of vaccines against a wide range of microbes. They also explore the basic mechanisms responsible for bactoinfection and its use for the development of an HIV-1 vaccine.

THERAPEUTIC VACCINES FOR HIV-1 INFECTION

In keeping with the multidisciplinary nature of the IHV, the Vaccine, Clinical, and Basic Science Divisions are developing therapeutic vaccines for HIV-1 infection. Effective vaccines are designed to restore the immune suppression caused by HIV-1 by reducing circulating levels of the HIV-1 protein and Tat and interferon. Such vaccines might interfere with HIV replication since they require Tat.

MOLECULAR ENDOCRINOLOGY

Bruce Weintraub, M.D., Head of the Laboratory of Molecular Endocrinology, conducts structure–function studies of glycoprotein hormones and growth factors.[5] These studies will determine

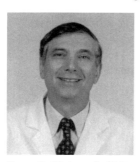

Bruce D. Weintraub, M.D.
Professor, Medicine
(Endocrinology)

those facets of these compounds or their receptors that can be changed to enhance their usefulness. This information is needed to design drugs rationally rather than use the traditional inefficient and haphazard screening techniques for new therapeutic regimens. Weintraub's findings will prove useful in virologic systems because glycoproteins comprise the capsids of many viruses. This includes HIV-1 and glycoprotein receptors, which are often used by viruses to gain entrance into the cell. Weintraub synthesized a "superhormone" version of thyroid-stimulating hormone that is 1–10,000 times more active than its natural analog. This should prove useful for diagnosis and treatment of thyroid cancer.

Paola Secchiero, Ph.D., and David Margolis, M.D., in the Clinical and Basic Research Divisions, are clarifying how HHV-6 might influence the progression of HIV-1 mechanisms and how repression of HIV-1 transcription is regulated.

KAPOSI'S SARCOMA

Another major research focus that employs the resources of all the IHV divisions is Kaposi's sarcoma (KS) pathogenesis. This research, conducted primarily by Gallo, Bryant, William Reid, D.V.M., Felipe Samaniego, M.D., and Lunardi-Iskandar, indicates that KS requires infection with HHV-8, and HIV-1 plays a catalytic role in HHV-8 infections by increasing the production of inflammatory cytokines.[6,7] Marvin Reitz, Ph.D., and Sandra Colombini, M.D., in addition, are conducting studies aimed at elucidating the HHV-9 genes that play a role in the oncogenesis of KS malignant tumors.[8]

Critical to the KS studies were the animal models developed by Gallo, Bryant, and Reid. KS tumors do not spontaneously develop in animals, nor can they be induced by viral infections. They established a KS animal model by transplanting human KS tumors into immunodeficient mice. The IHV's Animal Models Division has developed other innovative animal models for chronic infections such as AIDS and AIDS-related diseases including an HIV rat. Although laboratory rats are inexpensive and easily utilized, they are not readily infected with HIV. Using transgenic techniques, Bryant and Reid created a rat AIDS animal model. This will prove useful for unraveling the pathogenesis and treatment for AIDS and AIDS-associated diseases.

BREAST CANCER

Priscilla Furth, M.D., is studying breast cancer by uniquely evaluating the natural disappearance of breast cells after breast-feeding ceases.[9] She hopes to adapt this process—known as involution—to breast cancer. By observing involution in genetically engineered mice in the IHV's Animal Core Facility, she pinpoints those compounds which kill breast cancer cells.

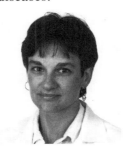

Priscilla A. Furth, M.D.
Assoc. Prof. Of Medicine

PFISTERIA

David Oldach, M.D., has challenged Chesapeake Bay's most pressing current biologic problem: identification of toxins in Pfiesteria, an organism that is presumably responsible for overwhelming fish kills and causing human illness in the mid-Atlantic region.[10] Oldach and colleagues around the world are developing a rapid and specific DNA analy-

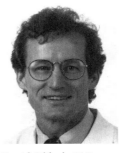

David Oldach, M.D.
Asst. Prof., Medicine

sis test to detect Pfiesteria and other toxic microorganisms in estuaries. He was one of the few initial medical authorities who reported such Pfiesteria-related symptoms as short-term memory loss.

VACCINE TRIALS

In the IHV's Epidemiology and Prevention Division, epidemiologist Farley Cleghorn, M.D., M.P. H., and his colleagues are conducting vaccine preparedness and Phase II clinical tests of an AIDS vaccine in Trinidad.[11] This country is afflicted with the same HIV-1 subtype predominant in the United States. International research by Alash'le Abimiku, Ph.D., is documenting the HIV strains prevalent in Nigeria and how their pathogenesis differs from HIV-1 subtype B. She is also assessing how Nigerian strains interact with chemokines and chemokine receptors and what the natural immunity to those strains is in Nigerians. In animal studies, Abimiku will assess the various HIV strains prevalent in Nigeria and how effective current HIV-1 vaccines are in promoting biologic protection from those strains.[12] Vaccine preparedness studies in Nigeria, where one-fifth of Africa's population resides, will also be included.

CLINICAL CARE OF HIV

Lori Fantry, M.D., M.P.H., is the medical director of the Evelyn Jordan Center, an AIDS clinic associated with the IHV and the University of Maryland Medical Center. With Charles Davis of the Clinical Research and Care Division at the IHV, Fantry is responsible for providing quality care to patients with complicated infectious diseases and coordinating clinical trials in the Institute facility.[13] The Institute's clinical care program encompasses numerous external facilities, including:

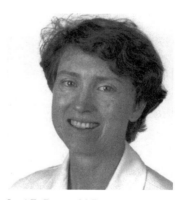

Lori E. Fantry, M.D.
Asst. Prof., Medicine

- outpatient HIV care
- a women's center
- inpatient care, palliative care
- home health
- hospice care

One entire floor of the Institute has comprehensive research laboratories, clinical diagnostic facilities, and a clinical research center with classrooms and patient examination rooms.

Dr. Kris A. Oursler former house officer in Medicine (1992–95) works productively on clinical and epidemiological factors related to pathogenesis of HIV infections including seroconverters and their relationship to immunotherapy.

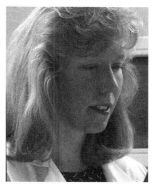

Kris Ann Oursler, M.D.
Asst. Prof., Medicine

Members of the Institute function regularly as instructors in the Educational and Teaching Conferences at the Medical School and University Hospital. They attend on the medical wards and patient clinics by rendering patient care, and as mentors for medical students and house officers. Their attendance and participation during regular weekly seminars and grand rounds adds greatly to the medical and research information provided by such teaching sessions.

REFERENCES

1. Cocchi F, DeVico AL, Garzino-Demo A, Arya SK, Gallo RC, Lusso P. Identification of RANTES, MIP-1, alpha, and MIP-1 beta as the major HIV-suppressive factors produced by CD8 + T cells. Science 1995;270(5243):1811–1815.

2. Lunardi-Iskandar Y, Bryant JL, Blattner WA, Hung CL, Flamand L, Gill P, Hermans P, Birken S, Gallo RC. Effects of a urinary factor from women in early pregnancy on HIV-1, SIV and associated disease. Nat Med 1998;4(4):428–434.

3. Wu S, Pascual DW, Lewis GK, Hone DM. Induction of mucosal and systemic responses against human immunodeficiency virus type 1 glycoprotein 120 in mice after oral immunization with a single dose of a

Salmonella-HIV vector. AIDS Res Hum Retroviruses 1997;13(14): 1187–1194.

4. Hone DM, Wu S, Powell RJ, Pascual DW, Van Cott J, McGhee J, Fouts TR, Tuskan RG, Lewis GK. Optimization of live oral Salmonella-HIV-1 vaccine vectors for the induction of HIV-specific mucosal and systemic immune responses. J Biotechnol 1996;44(1–3):203–207.

5. Grossman M, Leitolf H, Weintraub BD, Szkudlinski MW. A rational design strategy for protein hormone superagonists. Nat Biotechnol 1998;16(9):871–875.

6. Samaniego F, Pintus A, Gallo RC, Ensoli B. Vascular endothelial growth factor and basic fibroblast growth factor present in Kaposi's sarcoma (KS) are inducted by inflammatory cytokines and synergize to promote vascular permeability and KS lesion development. Am Pathol 1998;152(6):1433–1443.

7. Samaniego F, Markham PD, Gendelman R, Gallo RC, Ensoli B. Inflammatory cytokines induce endothelial cells to produce and release basic fibroblast growth factor and to promote Kaposi's sarcoma-like lesions in nude mice. J Immunol 1997;158(4):1887–94.

8. Guo HG, Browning P, Nicholas J, Hayward GS, Tschachler E, Jiang YW, Sadowska M, Raffeld M, Colombini S, Gallo RC, Reitz MS Jr. Characterization of a chemokine receptor-related gene in human herpes virus 8 and its expression in Kaposi's sarcoma. Virology 1997; 228(2):371–378.

9. Furth PA. SV40 rodent tumor models as paradigms of human disease: Transgenic mouse models. Dev Biol Stand 1998;94:281–287.

10. Golub JE, Haselow DT, Hageman JC, Lopez AS, Oldach DW, Grattan LM, Perl TM. Pfiesteria in Maryland: Preliminary epidemiologic findings. Md Med J 1998;47(3):137–143.

11. Cleghorn FR, Jack N, Murphy JR, Edwards J, Mahabir B, Paul R, O'Brien T, Greenberg M, Weinhold K, Bartholomew C. Brookmeyer R, Blattner WA. Direct and indirect estimates of HIV-1 incidence in a high-prevalence population. Am J Epidemiol 1998;147(90):834–839.

12. Abimiku AG, Frnachini G, Tartaglia J, Aldrich K, Myagkikh M, Markham PD, Chong P, Klein M, Kieny MP, Paoletti E, et al. HIV-1 recombinant poxvirus vaccine induces cross-protection against HIV-2 challenge in rhesus macaques. Nat Med 1995;1(4):321–329.

13. Fantry L, Tramont EC. Treatment of early syphilis. N Engl J Med 1997;337(23):1697–1698.

22

ESTABLISHMENT OF INTERNATIONAL CENTER FOR MEDICAL RESEARCH AND TRAINING (ICMRT)

Theodore E. Woodward, M.D.

In 1959, the Congress, through the Department of State and the National Institutes of Health (NIH), decided to establish a few selected centers designed to strengthen the discipline of tropical or global medicine in certain U.S. medical institutions and through them establish a scientific center in a foreign country. These were called ICMRT (International Centers for Medical Research and Training). Funds were set aside in the amount of 5 million dollars for such activities and a similar amount each year for an indefinite period. Solicitation under NIH sponsorship was completed and, ultimately, five such centers were authorized: University of California, Tulane University Medical Center, Louisiana State Medical University, The Johns Hopkins Medical Institutions, and the University of Maryland School of Medicine.

An initial invitation was made to our University through Dr. Joseph E. Smadel and Dr. James A. Shannon, Deputy Director and Director of the National Institutes of Health, respectively. Maryland's proposal, which comprised planning by the Division of Infectious Diseases of the Department of Medicine and the De-

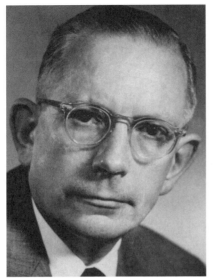

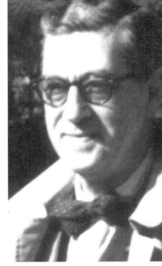

Joseph E. Smadel, M.D.   *James H. Shannon, M.D.*

partment of Microbiology, was formulated, and the University was ultimately successful in obtaining a grant.

Obviously, the choice and subsequent acceptance of a foreign site was a major issue. It was absolutely essential that the University of Maryland possess the professional personnel with strong interests in public health and preventive medicine. Equally important was the ready approval by the host country which not only needed a program, but which desired the acceptance of an outside visitor such as the United States. In other words, *need* and *desire* by either party were essential, with clear acknowledgment that a long-term commitment was necessary to ensure that key professional personnel would not only grow in stature, but simultaneously contribute significantly to improvement of better health preventive medicine and health practices in that country. U.S. authorities needed to ensure recruitment of young, as well as experienced, personnel who could develop new knowledge and capability to study the relevant diseases prevalent in that country, as well as those of global significance.

West Pakistan appeared to be a very desirable site. In East Pakistan (now Bangladesh), the Dacca Program in Cholera, which began in 1960, was progressing rapidly and producing rich rewards. Very crucial to the success of a foreign research and training program was the high prevalence of the various infections and nutritionally related diseases in the host countries, ripe for study. Pakistan very favorably fulfilled this requirement. Health officials in West Pakistan were very receptive to development of a joint program in their environment. Their material resources were partially available for development, including laboratory and administrative facilities. This was contingent upon the availability of necessary resources needed for organization, renovation, and recruitment of necessary personnel. Quite relevant at this time was Pakistan's membership in our government's SEATO Program (South-East Asia Treaty Organization).

The award was made to the Departments of Medicine and Microbiology with Doctors Fred McCrumb and Charles L. Wisseman as codirectors. These centers were conceived to advance the studies of the health sciences in the United States and in other countries, thereby stimulating research and improving health. They were regarded as cooperative enterprises in health, research, and training, and provided suitable laboratory and clinical facilities and appropriate professional staff at Maryland and abroad. Our activities included problems of nutrition, enteric diseases, malaria, fevers of obscure origin, demography, rickettsioses, and meningitis.

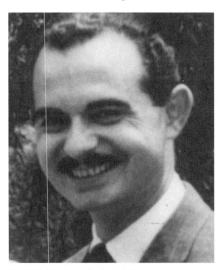

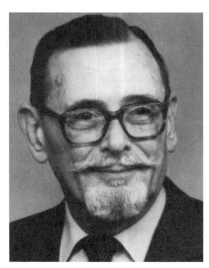

Fred R. McCrumb, Jr., M.D.   *Charles L. Wisseman, Jr., M.D.*

Dr. Colin M. MacLeod, a distinguished biologist and respected governmental advisor, assisted in development of the ICMRT program on several occasions. Memorable is our long train ride from Karachi through the long and hot Sind and Punjab provinces to Lahore for an exploratory visit. One stop during the two-day trip was at Multan, where Alexander the Great sustained his last serious wound when he led his forces over the fortress walls to subdue his adversary. With this wound, this great general began his downfall. The temperature in Multan on the day we visited was 115°F.

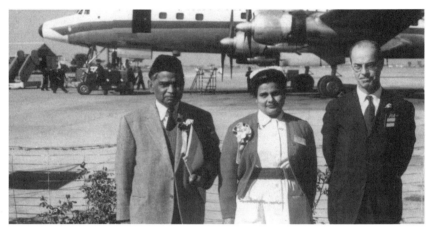

Minister of Health, Chief Matron, Colin MacLeod—Lahore 1962

On arrival at Lahore Station late the evening of the second day, we were weary, distraught, and wondered where we would find a bed. The American Consul, Mr. Andrew Corry, a Montanian by birth, had noted our presence in Pakistan; he had dispatched his aide to the station and took us in. He was a dedicated American diplomat who gave us much relevant assistance. He advised us to place the Research and Training Center in Lahore, the cultural center of old India. His advice was to locate sufficiently distant from the West Pakistan government and military center, then in Rawalpindi, to avoid interference, but to remain sufficiently close and in contact with the central government to avoid being forgotten. This was ultimately accomplished. The Center Building was newly planned and constructed at nominal cost, adjacent to the long established, but mostly unused, school of Public Health, in the central area of Lahore on Jail Road. Our neighbors and new friends gave wise administrative and intellectual help.

These modern laboratories opened for work in June 1963, and provided facilities for a large clinical ward and the utilization of a unit health center serving a large native population. Dr. Merrill J. Snyder spent the Summer of 1962 directing the installation of the new laboratories.

Dr. Eugene Gangarosa was the first Director of our Center in Lahore beginning in 1962. He was innovative and established many important institutional relationships which were of great assistance in developing a scientific and training program. Dr. Herbert Barnett, Chief Entomologist, next served as Director. In 1964, it fell to my lot to direct the Lahore ICMRT. By this time, there was a full decade of Chairmanship of Medicine behind me in Baltimore, a talented and dedicated faculty were hard at work there, and it seemed reasonable that a break to help shore up things in Lahore was advisable. The Dean and university administration granted a sabbatical leave, provided I found supportive salary funds for the leave. This was accomplished, and the appointment was approved by the NIH. Dr. John Wiswell served most effectively as Acting Chairman of the Department of Medicine in Baltimore during the interim. Dr. Richard Baker joined the program in 1966–1967, and directed the Pakistan Medical Research Center (PMRC) program in Lahore in 1971–1979. From 1967 to 1971 Dr. Baker and Dr. Richard Sakai were interim directors. Dr. David Nalin succeeded him from 1979–1981; Dr. Thomas Strickland became Director in 1981.

Dr. Nur Ahmad, former Commandant of the Armed Forces Institute of Pathology, Rawalpindi, was appointed to the faculty. He coordinated the Pakistan program and served as the pathologist for the unit. Dr. Christian R. Klimt was appointed as Chief Epidemiologist.

The ICMRT Programs always had pro-

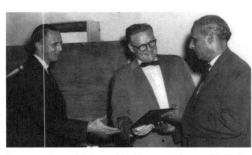

Presentation of Library Dedicatory Plaque (PMRC) to Dr. Nur Ahmad by Dr. Richard Mason

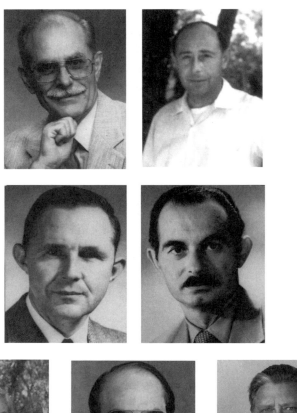

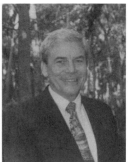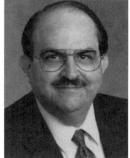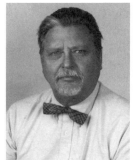

Directors of the ICMRT: Eugene J. Gangorosa, M.D. (1962–1963); Herbert C. Barnett, Ph.D. (1963–1964); Theodore E. Woodward, M.D. (1964–1965); Fred R. McCrumb, Jr., M.D. (1965–1966); Richard H. Baker, Ph.D. (1966–1967, 1971–1979); David R. Nalin, M.D. (1979–1981); G. Thomas Strickland, M.D. (1981–1995)

fessional medical personnel from the host country whose knowledge and experience with local disease problems and health practices were essential for ensuring stability and maintaining governmental relationships. Recruitment was accomplished at all professional levels. Pakistan regulations required that salary scales be adjusted to local rather than U.S.A. standards, with fringe benefits added as indicated. When Pakistani personnel served in the United States, University of Maryland salary scales were to be applied.

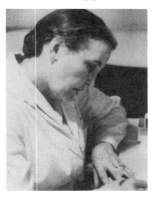

Celeste Woodward, M.D., my wife, geared up for her contribution. She spent endless hours of study and working clinical sessions in Baltimore to bone up on internal medicine and the important discipline of dermatology.

Arriving in Lahore, we were met at the air terminal and promptly taken to our quarters which were delightful. Our residence for the next 10 months was a lovely, small one-floor villa in Shah Jamal with very adequate space and a lovely garden. Furthermore, qualified servants to perform household chores were available, being passed on to us by departing American residents.

Celeste Woodward, M.D.

The research and training center, known as the University of Maryland Pakistan Medical Research Center (PMRC), was well organized and centrally located. The city was one of contrasts. The daily life and customs are similar to those of centuries ago. In the country, the ways and customs date to biblical times. Yet,

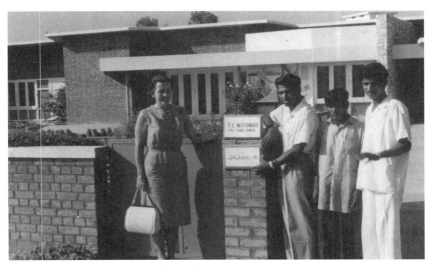

Residence: Shah Jamal, Lahore. Celeste Woodward, Abdul, Sardar, and Ali.

in Lahore there are also modern developments which will rival any urban settings in America.

ICMRT RESEARCH ACTIVITIES

The unique opportunity to study new control methods for malaria in the highly endemic area of West Pakistan prompted the initiation of a multifaceted malaria research program. The program included field evaluation of cycloguanil, the dihydrothiazine metabolite of chlorguanide, CI-501 (Parke-Davis and Company) and the fumigant insecticide DDVP. In addition, emphasis was placed on the study of immune mechanisms in malaria and the occurrence of drug-resistance strains of human plasmodia.

A broad research program on the rickettsial diseases of Pakistan was initiated under the direction of Dr. C.L. Wisseman, Jr., Professor and Head, Department of Microbiology. The long-term objectives of the study included investigation of the types, distribution, various ecologies, and medical importance of the rickettsioses of West Pakistan among human populations. The initial project was an ecologic study of scrub typhus. The investigation showed that small mammals serving as vertebrate hosts were abundant and widely distributed in West Pakistan. *Rickettsia tsutsugamushi* was isolated from human beings, rodents, and ectoparasites, confirming the importance of this area as a reservoir of infection.

Studies on the bionomics of mosquitoes as related to arthropod-borne viruses and malaria were undertaken in the Lahore area in 1962. During the course of this project, it was demonstrated that the risk of exposure of humans to vector mosquitoes in general was uncommon in the urban areas, thereby reducing the likelihood of acquiring malaria in Lahore. *Aedes* (Stegomyia) species were common, suggesting the possibility that dengue virus may be present. Rural collections revealed the prevalence of *Culex tritaeniorhynchus* and *Anopheles culicifacies* vectors of West Nile virus and malaria, respectively.

Antibody studies among inhabitants of the Lahore area also revealed the presence of Group B arthropod-borne viruses, sandfly fever, Q fever, and other rickettsioses and brucellosis. The high prevalence of enteroviral antibodies was in keeping with reports from similar environments in other newly developing nations.

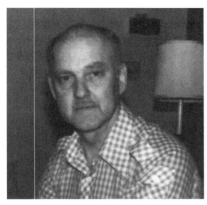

Michael B. Gregg, M.D.

Dr. Michael B. Gregg, a Case Western Reserve medical graduate, joined our department as a research associate in the ICMRT Program in 1962. Mike was quite interested in immunology and the application of serologic techniques as diagnostic aids. He was Assistant Professor of Medicine and Director of the Division of Serology in the Lahore, Pakistan Program from 1963 to 1966. Later, he made a remarkable record with the CDC Program in Atlanta; he headed the Viral Diseases Division there for 10 years, and was Editor of the *CDC Morbidity/Mortality Report* for 21 years and Director of the Epidemiology Program.

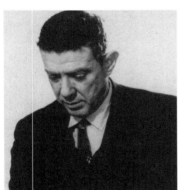

Robert Traub, M.D., Ph.D.

Dr. Robert Traub contributed importantly to the ICMRT Program in Pakistan beginning in 1965. Pioneering studies showed that interpretation of faunal data allowed accurate prediction of prevalence of certain ectoparasite-borne diseases in foci or geographic sites where their prior existence was either not expected or unknown. This exhaustive evaluation ultimately revealed scrub and tick typhus in semi-deserts, mountain deserts, and subarctic mountain terrain in Pakistan.[1-3] Traub's innovative studies and findings led to formulation of the concept that humans acquire zoonotic infections such as plague, tularemia, and anthrax from those animals higher in the evolutionary scale, such as rodents or hoofed animals, rather than from lower forms like marsupials or insectivores.[4]

Mohammed A. Aziz, a 1954 graduate of the Dacca Medical College received his doctoral degree from the University of Minnesota in 1962, specializing in clinical pathology and porphyrin metabolism. He joined the ICMRT Program in 1962 as a research associate with work at the PMRC, Lahore. He progressed through the faculty ranks to associate professor in 1967 and as Head of the Division of Clinical Investigation at the PMRC. He was Associate Director of the Center from 1967 to 1973. Aziz had broad capabilities, and his published work embraced etiology, pathogenesis and control of enteric infections, hepatitis, bilirubin metabolism, and anemia. Dr. Aziz later became Director for Domestic Clinical Research at Merck, Sharpe and Dohme in 1976, and Senior

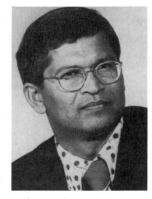

Mohammed A. Aziz, M.D., Ph.D.

Director for International Clinical Research in 1981. He became recognized nationally and internationally as a tropical medicine authority, particularly with respect to the importance of anti-infective drugs such as Ivermectin in onchocerciasis.

Fatima Begum Aziz, M.S., Ph.D., received her doctorate in virology from the London School of Hygiene and Tropical Medicine in 1963. She joined the ICMRT Program in 1964 and until 1970, while a faculty member in microbiology, she contributed productively in arthro-borne viral infections and encephalitis at the PMRC, Lahore and in Baltimore. From 1966 to 1968, she served as a postdoctoral fellow at the University of Maryland with training in 1967 at the Yale Arbovirus Research Unit and the National Center for Disease Control in Atlanta in 1968.

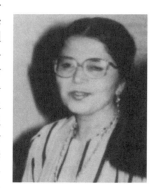

Fatima Begum Aziz, M.S., Ph.D.

PROGRAM IN MEDICINE IN DERMATOLOGY

Celeste was taken in almost immediately at the Fatima Jinnah College which was solely for women students. Single-handedly, she established and organized a dermatology clinic which steadily grew in numbers once started. She devoted about equal time at the King Edward Medical College which was coeducational. Daily she came home with stories of having detected cases of leprosy (which was believed not to be prevalent in Lahore), cutaneous leishmaniasis (a protozoal disease), scabies, psoriasis, and contact dermatitis caused by too much and unnecessary treatment. There were hosts of other disorders. Immediately she made a name for herself and the medical center. Frequently, she was called for consultations, by both the affluent and the impoverished. As a woman physician, she could examine other women thoroughly, something denied to male dermatologists. Her friend, Dr. Ghulam Shabbir, would say, "kindly tell me what the lesion looks like since I have never seen it." His earlier training in dermatology had been taken in England, yet this menagerie of skin disorders in Pakistan was limitless. Celeste was kept very busy, and when we left, her departure left a dent in the dermatologic services, particularly the one at Fatima Jinnah which she had so devotedly and efficiently developed.

Her star patient was a most grateful Mian Said Siagol, an intelligent and most successful industrialist. He had unfortunately been treated excessively with radiation therapy for common warts located in a sensitive anatomical area. Skin necrosis and wide inflammation had produced a horrible reaction. There was initial reluctance on the part of family and house personnel to accept a woman physician. Yet, she carefully and authoritatively took over and in a few days her treatment had produced striking results. She was quickly taken into the family confidence and even the guard at the entrance of one of his many mansions came to attention when she approached. We were entertained at dinner on a memorable occasion with the entire family—children, grandchildren, and several of his wives—in attendance, all served at a huge table. The dinner, out of *Arabian Nights*, was elaborate and delicious. Following dinner, Celeste was presented with a delicately tooled, wide gold bracelet imbedded with many precious and semi-precious stones which, we understand, had been a part of his first wife's wedding gifts.

My chores were a bit different. We had young physicians and technical staff members of the research center who needed guidance, discipline, and assistance. The laboratory research facilities were primitive and needed modernization. There was no library; time moved less rapidly and patience was necessary in awaiting replenishment from the States. I purchased a slide projector and microscope in Tokyo rather than wait for another through normal requisition procedures. On several occasions, it was necessary to provide personal funds to meet the laboratory payroll. Communications with Baltimore were often erratic. Yet, we made it.

Before going to Lahore, my clinical interests had prompted me to seek an academic appointment to the two Lahore medical schools, the King Edward and Fatima Jinnah Medical Colleges. This was ultimately accomplished through the good offices of Dr. Gene Gangarosa and Dr. Andrew Corry, American Consul General. I was granted a Visiting Professorship in each of these schools which took time to accomplish and was not a routine practice.

Accompanying us to Lahore were Dr. Allan Ronald and his wife Myrna and Dr. Larry Gallagher and his wife Anne. Ronald and Gallagher were programmed to do special work on infectious diseases, and my faculty appointment opened doors for clinical studies since I was given immediate assignment to teach medical students on ward rounds. These started at 7:00 a.m., and it was cold during the winter months. Much of the teaching was with small groups of about 10 each, every other day from 7:00 a.m. until noon. It was purely clinical, history taking, physical examination, and clinical interpretation. Laboratory backup was almost nonexistent, which, at times, is not a bad system at all. Most of the physical examinations stopped at the navel, but we changed that, at least in men. I taught them sigmoidoscopy—much to the consternation of everyone. Amoebic dysentery and bacillary dysentery are very common in tropical countries, and examination of the lower intestine is essential for proper interpretation. Students and junior registrars (medical residents) were delighted to learn something new.

I arranged for a local craftsman to take my sigmoidoscope and make a half dozen duplicates, silverplated, calibrated better than the original, for the sum of 12 rupees ($6) each. The original cost for one in 1948 was $35.00. A complete sigmoidoscopic set with a light system was given to each medical service on which I attended. During my stay, they were used, but after our departure, these units blended into oblivion.

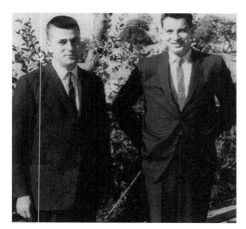

Larry Gallagher, M.D., and Allan R. Ronald, M.D.

These were great clinical times. Allan Ronald and Larry Gallagher studied febrile patients of all types: typhoid fever, amoebic dysentery, liver abscess, leptospirosis, malaria, endemic infections, and many others. We were able to develop a special clinical ward for the study of typhoid in a municipal hospital just outside Lahore. Several clinical disorders, new to Pakistan, were detected through these studies.

OBSCURE FEVER (FUO)

In a study of febrile diseases in hospitalized patients in the Lahore area, a systematic study was made to identify those diseases whose nature was not apparent at the time of initial examination. It was assumed that a comprehensive evaluation would provide helpful guidelines for the medical profession relative to incidence and uncover new infectious agents, heretofore unrecognized. Table 1 lists the confirmed clinical diagnoses of 357 patients whose fever lasted three weeks or less; Table 2 provides data on 28 patients febrile for three or more weeks. Table 3 lists the newly identified infectious diseases detected in West Punjab, 1964–1966.

AMOEBIC LIVER ABSCESS

In 10 patients with single hepatic amoebic abscesses, helpful bedside clues to localization were: 1) an obvious bulge of the lower chest wall, upper abdomen, and prominence of intercostal interspaces; 2) presence of hepatic friction rub; and 3) elevation of the diaphragm on the right with a high dull percussion impulse confirmed by a lateral roentgenogram. Biopsy of intact rectosigmoid mucosa frequently revealed amoeba when fecal specimens were negative.

Table 1.   Clinical Diagnoses of 357 Patients with Fever of Three Weeks or Less

Enteric group	
Typhoid	78
Salmonelloses	16
Dysentery	6
Respiratory	
Pneumonia, lobar	12
Pneumonia, viral	19
Viral U.R.I.	102
Meningoencephalitis	
Viral	5
Pyogenic	16
Hepatic group	
Hepatitis, viral	4
Abscess, amoebic	3
Viral group	
Enterovirus	11
Parotitis, orchitis	4
Variola	1
Other	42
Miscellaneous	
Malaria, leptospirosis, typhus, pharyng, hem. anemia	13
Undiagnosed	11
	357

COMMUNITY MALARIA STUDIES

Malaria has always ravaged Asian people, and this mosquito-borne illness was very prevalent in the Punjab. Our research interests were directed at identifying the types of malaria prevalent, the mosquitoes transmitting them, and evaluation of vector control by attacking mosquitoes. A new technique involved the placing of small, vinyl, plastic-like strips impregnated with an anti-mosquito chemical agent in village huts. A number of villages north of Lahore were made available for our use, and it was possible to make studies in a village with the vinyl strips as a control. Samples of blood were taken by finger stick on a regular basis, and spleens were palpated, since the splenic index of enlargement is a good marker for the presence of malaria.

Table 2. Clinical Diagnoses of 28 Patients Whose Febrile Course
Exceeded Three Weeks

Infectious diseases	
Tuberculosis	10
Brucellois	1
Abscess, Liver	7
Abscess,	1
Retroperitoneal	1
Cholangitis	1
Endocarditis	2
Consective tissue diseases	
S.L.E.	2
Rheumatic fever	1
Neoplastic diseases	
Lymphoma	1
Hepatoma	1
Miscellaneous	
Factitious	1
	28

NUTRITIONAL STUDIES

Dr. Barbara Underwood worked creatively on malnutrition problems, which were so prevalent throughout rural Pakistan in northern villages. The broad objective was to evaluate the relationship between nutrition, dietary habits, incidence of infection, and growth of preschool Pakistani children, who were most vul-

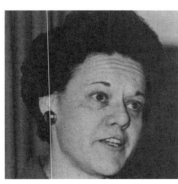

Barbara A. Underwood, M.D., Ph.D.

nerable to nutritional diseases and infection. Her work blended closely with the malaria study program. She established warm relationships with village Pakistani women, spoke their language, and wore their native dress. She collected and evaluated mother's milk during the lactation period and established that it was remarkably deficient in necessary nutrients. Often Buffalo milk was used for those who could afford it. Her work led to recom-

Table 3.   Newly Identified Infections in West Punjab, 1964–1966 (ICMRT)

Respiratory	*Enteric*
Influenza virus	ECHO
A.B.C.	Coxsackie
Respiratory syncytial	
Parainfluenza 1.3	
Adenovirus	*Rickettsial*
Mycoplasma	Tick-borne typhus
Arbovirus	Scrub typhus
Dengue	Q fever
West Nile	*Miscellaneous*
Sandfly fever	Leptospirosis
	Psittacosis

mended dietary changes in the standard basic diet of chipati (un-leavened wheat bread).

HEMOLYTIC ANEMIA

Of special interest was finding four patients with hemolytic ane-mia manifested by fever, dark urine (hemoglobinuria), and severe anemia, having hemolyzed about 80% of their erythrocytes. Each patient showed a deficiency of glucose-6-phosphate dehydroge-nase in their erythrocytes. They had previously received either primaquine or quinacrine for malaria or sulfone tablets, in one, for a skin lesion. All four patients recovered. A limited survey in approximately 500 students and military personnel in West Pa-kistan revealed an incidence of this enzyme defect in about 2%. This was a new finding to West Pakistan.

A pleasant part of our Lahore experience was receiving visi-tors and friends from the United States. Dr. William (Bill) Mos-berg, an able Baltimore neurosurgeon, came to Lahore from Karachi where he had consulted for USAID. Dr. James Steele, a prominent veterinary scientist and educator, came with his son for a few days. He was en route to India where he was to advise about contraceptive devices for cattle which caused this large Asian country considerable trouble. Charley and Ann McCormick broke their round-the-world trip at Bombay and came to Lahore for a few days. We had a great time showing them the sights, such as the Bad Shaii Mosque and Red Fort in

Lahore, Kim's Cannon, "Zam Zammah," on the mall just across from the museum, the old city, and Jehangir's Tomb just outside Lahore to the north. We accompanied them to Delhi and with them visited the Taj Mahal in Agra which was a special treat for everyone.

Lahore, a very interesting city, was one of the cultural centers of India in the early days of Mogul rulers. Rudyard Kipling spent many of his most productive and happy years in this capital of the Punjab. During the imperialistic days of the British Raj, the Lahore Officers Club on Shahrae Quaid-E-Azam avenue was a center of social life. When our Pakistan program began, Dr. David Clyde was Director of the Malaria Program in Baltimore, actively involved in testing new vaccines and promising chemotherapeutic drugs. His father, Maj. Gen. David Clyde (later Sir) was Inspector General, Civil Hospitals, the Punjab (including Pakistan and Indian Sections) based at Lahore during World War II. He became Surgeon General, Bengal, from the end of the war until Independence in 1947. He received his knighthood in the "Dissolutions Honors" list. His portrait was prominently displayed in the Lahore Officers' Club.

In early January 1965, Colin MacLeod, then with the Office of Science and Technology of the White House, cabled an invitation for me to join a small working group as an official delegate in Tokyo to help develop a joint U.S.-Japanese Medical Science Program. This was gratefully accepted and soon I was briefly associated with Colin, Jim Shannon (Director of NIH), Thomas Francis (University of Michigan, Preventive Medicine), Jack Weir (Rockefeller Foundation), and Stanley Bennett (University North Carolina). We met first at the American Embassy in Tokyo and later with Japanese scientists to inaugurate the U.S.–Japan Cooperative Medical Science Program which has contributed importantly to the control of tuberculosis, leprosy, encephalitis, cholera, schistosomiasis, filariasis, and other infectious diseases so prevalent in Southeast Asian countries. The program remains viable and productive, and in its 33rd year, its scientific scope has been extended. It is a model of bi-national cooperation.

Numerous festive occasions added greatly to this interesting period in West Pakistan. Weddings usually were planned for the autumn when the weather was more agreeable. Houses, trees, and bushes were gaily decorated with colorful electric lights and bright decorations of all kinds. At night, they resembled a huge Christmas garden. Weddings were segregated and, on arriving, men were ushered into a huge tent where conversation went on for hours. The beverage was usually a lime or orange squash, a shock to many Westerners. After awhile, this experience was interrupted by band and trumpet music which announced arrival of the groom. He, along with his father or brother, was met by the bride's father and brother who came to the men's reception area where the marriage agreement was signed and witnessed. These agreements in addition to providing dowries to support the newlyweds also set the responsibilities and rights of the bride and groom and their families.

The ladies had a much happier time. They were gaily dressed and were shown the various lovely wedding gifts which, I understand, always came in pairs. Indeed, the bride's dressing was often helped by guests and friends. Then a special dramatic event occurred unwitnessed by the men. The bridegroom, if this was a fully orthodox wedding ceremony, had never seen his bride. The marriage was usually arranged by family—a favorite uncle always looked out for his nephew. The groom was led to the ladies' tent, blindfolded, and placed in a chair. The marriage chair is low with the seat several inches off the ground. The bride was also seated, blindfolded in a similar chair, being separated from the groom by a partition so that they could not see each other. Then, at a crucial moment, blindfolds were removed and each looked forward to a mirror which would allow the first glance. I mentioned to Celeste that the low chair was a good idea because if he had a sudden attack of syncope, he did not have far to fall! The nuptials were then followed by buffets in separate tents, male and female.

A particularly happy assignment for me was a visit every other week to Rawalpindi to give lectures to officers and ancillary health personnel of the Armed Forces Medical School. Mornings were spent in the ward walks with the opportunity to see and discuss many interesting cases—including typhoid fever, amoebic liver abscess, meningitis, encephalitis, and malaria. Cases were clearly and formally presented. These rounds were followed by a lecture; indeed, a series of lectures were given over the eight-month period. I enjoyed the opportunity to have lunch

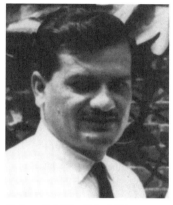

Zaheer Ud-Din, B.S., M.B.

in the Old Officers Club which used beautiful porcelain ware and decorative silver service. For about a decade after returning to Baltimore, the Surgeon General of the Pakistan Army selected a military officer who came to Maryland for a three-year period for training in internal medicine and a subspecialty of his choice. Three excellent officers came; the one who stood out was Zaheer Ud-Din, who made a hit with everyone in Baltimore. He later became the Surgeon General of Pakistan's Military Services.

When time came to pack and return home, we were confronted with a major problem. We had accumulated a number of household, artistic, and personal items which had to be crated. Celeste and Abdul handled most of this chore, which consisted of using small boxes which were then packed into a giant box. The resultant wooden crate was huge, as high as the house but not quite so broad. The carton was lifted mechanically to a van, and carted to the rail-line and ultimately to a ship in Karachi for surface transportation to Baltimore. Ultimately, we claimed it at the Custom House.

Following is a roster of former faculty members who made important contributions to the ICMRT Program including their faculty status and later career academic and administrative positions 1960–1980:

Ronald Anthony, M.D.
Asst. Prof., Pathology,
Univ. of Maryland

Mohammed A. Aziz, M.D.
Research Assoc., 1962, Asst.
Prof., Senior Director, Clinical
Research, Merck Research
Laboratories International

Richard H. Baker, Ph.D.
Prof. Microbiology, Univ. of
Maryland Director, ICMRT,
1971–1979, Director & Prof.,
Institute of Food &
Agricultural Sciences, Florida
Medical Entomology
Laboratory, University of
Florida

Herbert C. Barnett, Ph.D.
Assoc. Prof. Medicine, 1962,
Director, Division of Medical
Entomology, ICMRT

Frank A. Carozza, M.D.
Assoc. Prof. Medicine, Head,
Division of Introduction to
Medicine (Physical Diagnosis)
Medical Advisor, McCormick
& Co., Inc.

Eugene H. Gangarosa, M.D.
Asst. Prof., ICMRT,
1961–1964, Director, ICMRT,
1962–1964 Prof & Director,
Emory Univ., Dept. of
Community Health, Master,
Public Health Program,
Atlanta, Dean, American
University, Beirut

Michael B. Gregg, M.D.
Research Assoc., ICMRT,
1962–1964, Asst. Prof.,
1964–1966, Director, Division
Viral Diseases, CDC (10 yrs),
Editor, *Morbidity and
Mortality Reports* (21 yrs),
Director, Epidemiology, CDC,
Atlanta

Ashley Haase, M.D.
Prof. & Chair, Dept. of
Microbiology, Univ. of
Minnesota

Raymond Hepner, M.D.
Prof. & Acting Chairman,
Pediatrics, Univ. of Maryland
School of Medicine

Richard B. Hornick, M.D.
Prof. of Medicine & Head,
Division of Infectious Diseases,
Univ. of Maryland,
1963–1979, Prof. &
Chairman, Department of
Medicine, Univ. of Rochester
School of Medicine

Christian Klimt, M.D.
Assoc. Prof. Medicine, 1962;
Director, Division of
Epidemiology & Biostatistics,
ICMRT

Vincent C. McCarthy, M.D.
Asst. Prof., ICMRT, Medicine,
Microbiology, Director,
Insectory

Frederick R. McCrumb, Jr., M.D.
Prof. Medicine & Head,
Division of Infectious Diseases,
1958–1963, Co-Director,
ICMRT, Head, Division of
International Medicine

Gardner Middlebrook, M.D.
Staff member, Rockefeller
Institute, Prof. International
Medicine and Pathology,
Head, Division of Experimental
Pathology, Univ. of Maryland
School of Medicine

David Nalin, M.D.
Research Assoc., ICMRT,
Assoc. Prof., International
Medicine, Univ. of Maryland
School of Medicine, Director,
ICMRT 1979–1981, Director
of Clinical Research, Merck &
Co. Research Laboratories

Allan R. Ronald, M.D.
Chairman, Medical
Microbiology, Univ. of
Manitoba, Canada, Prof. &
Chairman, Dept. of Medicine,
University of Manitoba

Merrill J. Snyder, Ph.D.
Assoc. Prof. Medicine,
1949–1962, Prof. Experimental
Medicine, Univ. of Maryland
School of Medicine

Barbara A. Underwood, M.D.
Ph.D., Research Associate,
ICMRT, 1962, Assoc. Prof.,
Medicine, Univ. of Maryland,
Prof., Columbia School of
Public Health, Institute,
Nutritional Sciences, New York

Robert Traub, M.D., Ph.D.
Research Prof. of Medical
Microbiology, Univ. of
Maryland, 1962–1983,
Honorary Curator of Fleas,
Smithsonian Institute,
Washington, DC

Charles L. Wisseman, Jr., M.D.
Prof. & Chair, Depart. of
Microbiology & Immunology,
Univ. of Maryland 1954–1986

Celeste L. Woodward, M.D.
Asst. Prof. of Medicine, Univ.
of Maryland, 1964–1980,
AMA Volunteer Physician for
Refugees, Vietnam, Thailand,
1968, 1970, 1979, 1980

Theodore E. Woodward, M.D.
Prof. & Chairman, Dept. of
Medicine, 1954–1981, Prof.
Medicine Emeritus,
1981–present, Univ. of
Maryland School of Medicine,
Director, ICMRT, Lahore,
West Pakistan, 1964–1965

William E. Woodward, M.D.
Asst. Prof. Medicine, 1973,
Associate Professor of
Medicine, 1978–1979, Univ. of
Maryland School of Medicine,
Assoc. Prof. of Epidemiology,
Univ. of Texas School of Public
Health, 1979–1983, Medical
Director, McCormick & Co.,
Inc., Baltimore, 1983–1992

Zaheer Ud-Din, B.S., M.B.
Surgeon General, Pakistan
Medical Services

ICMRT LIST OF PUBLICATIONS

Aziz MA, Ahmad N, Path FC, Siddiqui AR. The lack of correlation between hookworm disease and intestinal malabsorption. Gastroenterology 1967;52:000.

Aziz MA, Siddiqui A. Congenital familial nonhemolytic hyperbilirubinemia in an adult with central nervous system derangement. Gastroenterology 1967;52:254–258.

Begum F. Langat virus: Differentiation of strains of reduced pathogenicity suitable for vaccines. Am J Trop Med Hyg 1969;6:18.

Begum F, Hoffman WW, Ackerman NR. Spontaneous motor activity and lung function during a non-lethal influenza infection in hamsters. Presented by W.W. Hoffman, Ph.D., October 27, 1976 at the 16th Science Conference on Antimicrobial Agents and Chemotherapy in Chicago.

Begum F, Wisseman CL, Casals J. Tick-borne viruses of West Pakistan. II. *Hazara* virus: a new agent isolated from Ixodes Redikorzevi ticks from the Kaghan Valley, West Pakistan. Am J Epidemiol 1970;92(3):192–4.

Begum F, Wisseman CL, Casals J. Tick-borne viruses of West Pakistan. III. Dera Ghase Khan virus: A new agent isolated from Hyalomma Dromedari ticks in the D.G. Karhn district of West Pakistan. Am J Epidemiol 1970;92(3):195–196.

Begum F, Wisseman CL, Casals J. Tick-borne viruses of West Pakistan. IV. Viruses similar to, or identical with, Crimean hemorrhagic fever (Congo-Semunya), Wad Medani and Pak Argas 461 isolated from ticks of the Changa Manga Forest Lahore District, and of Hunza Gilgit Agnecy, West Pakistan. Am J Epidemiol 1970;92(3):197–202.

Begum F, Wisseman CL, Traub R. Tick-borne viruses of West Pakistan. I. Isolation and general characteristics. Am J Epidemiol 1970;92(3):180–191.

Greisman SE, Carozza FA, Jr, Hills JD. Mechanisms of endotoxin tolerance. I. Relationship between tolerance and reticuloendothelial system phagocytic activity in the rabbit. J Exper Med 1963;117:663.

Greisman SE, Hornick RB, Carozza FA Jr, Woodward TE. Effect of endotoxin tolerance on human typhoid fever. Trans Assoc Am Physicians 1962;LXXV:170.

Greisman EE, Hornick RB, Carozza FA Jr, Woodward TE. The role of endotoxin during typhoid fever and tularemia in man:

Acquisition of tolerance to endotoxin. J Clin Invest 1963; 42:1062.

Greisman EE, Hornick RB, Carozza FA Jr, Woodward TE. Altered cardiovascular responses to catecholamines. J Clin Invest 1964;43:986.

Greisman SE, Hornick RB, Wagner HW Jr, Woodward TE. The integrity of the endotoxin tolerance mechanisms during typhoid fever in man. Trans Assoc Am Physicians 1967;LXXX:250.

Greisman SE, Hornick RB, Woodward TE. The role of endotoxin during typhoid fever and tularemia in man. III. Hyperreacitvity to endotoxin during infection. J Clin Invest 1964;43:1747.

Greisman SE, Wagner HN Jr, Lio M, Hornick RB. Mechanisms of endotoxin tolerance. II. Relationship between endotoxin tolerance and reticuloendothelial system phagocytic activity in man. J Exp Med 1964;119:241.

Greisman SE, Woodward WE. Mechanisms of endotoxin tolerance. III. The refractory state during continuous intravenous infusions of endotoxin. J Exp Med 1965;121:911.

Greisman SE, Young EJ, Woodward WE. Mechanisms of endotoxin tolerance. IV. Specificity of the pyrogenic refractory state during continuous intravenous infusions of endotoxin. J Exp Med 1966;124:983.

Hornick RB, Gallager LR, Ronald AR, Abdullah J, Khan MA, Khan I, Hassan S, Messer J, Shafi MJ, Ud-Din Z, Woodward TE. Chloramphenicol treatment of pyrogenic meningitis. Bull Sch Med Univ Maryland 1966;51:43.

Hornick RB, Woodward TE. Appraisal of typhoid vaccine in experimentally infected human subjects. Trans Am Clin Climatol Assoc 1966;78:70.

Hornick RB, Woodward TE, McCrumb FR, Snyder MJ, Dawkins AT, Bulkeley JT, de la Macorra F, Carozza FA. Study of induced typhoid fever in Man. I. Evaluation of vaccine effectiveness. Trans Assoc Am Phys 1966;LXXIX:361–367.

Hornick RB, Woodward TE, McCrumb FR, Snyder MJ, Dawkins AT, Bulkeley JT, de la Macorra F, Carozza FA. Typhoid fever vaccine—yes or no? Med Clin North America 1967;51:617.

Ronald AR, Underwood BA, Sadiqu Hasan, Basir MA, Gallagher LR, Naheed F, Khan M, Mallic SMK, Woodward TE. Primaquine-sensitive hemolytic anemia in West Pakistan. Pak J Med Res 1966;5(1):5–14.

Ronald AR, Underwood BA, Woodward TE. Glucose-6-phosphate dehydrogenase deficiency in Pakistani males. Trans R Soc Trop Med Hyg 1968;62:000.

Russell PK, Aziz N, Ahamn, Kent TH, Gangarosa E. Enteritis and gastritis in young asymptomatic Pakistani men. Am J Dig Disest 1996;11:196–302.

Russell PK, Bellanti JA, Buescher EL, McCown JM. Challenge virus resistance and interferon produced in BS-C-1 cells by dengue virus. Soc Exp Biol and Med 1966;122:557.

Russell PK, Buescher EL, McCown JO, Ordonez O. Recovery of dengue viruses from patients during epidemics in Puerto Rico and East Pakistan. A J Trop Med Hyg 1966;15:573.

Schubart AF, Hornick RB, Ewald RW, Schroeder WC, Myerburg RJ, Goodman JS, Woodward TE. Changes of serum complement of properdin levels in experimental typhoid fever, a longitudinal study of the disease including the incubation period and the phase of recovery following treatment with chloramphenicol. J Immunol 1964;93:367.

Shaffi MJ, Ud-Din Z, Woodward TE. Chloramphenicol treatment of pyrogenic meningitis. Bull Sch Med Univ Maryland 1966;51:43.

Snyder MJ, Dawkins AT, Bulkeley JT, de la Macorra F, Carozza FA: Typhoid fever vaccine-yes or no? Med Clin North Am 1967;51:617.

Snyder MJ, Hornick RB, McCrumb FR Jr, Morse LJ, Woodward TE. Asymptomatic typhoidal bacteremia in volunteers. Antimicrob Agents Chemother 1963;604–607.

Sprinz H, Gangarosa EJ, Williams M, Hornick RB, Woodward TE. Histopathology of the upper small intestines in typhoid fever. Biopsy study of experimental disease in man. Am J Digest Dis 1966;11:615–624.

Underwood BA, Hepner R, Cross E, Mirza AB, Haydt K, Kallue A. Height, weight and skin-fold thickness data collected during a survey of rural and urban populations of West Pakistan. Am J Clin Nutr 1967;20:694–701.

Wagner HN Jr, Ho M, Hornick RB. Studies of the reticuloendothelial system (RES). II. Changes in the phagocytic capacity of the RES in patients with certain infections. J Clin Invest 1963;42:427–434.

Woodward TE. Typhoid fever: A discussion of its pathogenesis, physiologic abnormalities and management. Trans Am Coll Physicians 1963;31:26.

Woodward TE. Research responsibilities in international health. Ann NY Acad Sci 1963;107:712–715.

Woodward TE, An American Clinician in Asia. Trans Coll Physician 1966;34:4.

Woodward TE. Typhoid in volunteers. Editorial. N Engl J Med 1968;278:332.

Woodward TE, Smadel JE. Management of typhoid fever and its complications. Ann Intern Med 1964;60:144.

Woodward TE, Terry LL. Research responsibilities in international health. Panel discussion. Ann NY Acad Sci 1963;107: 713.

Woodward TE, Woodward WE. The role of endotoxin during typhoid fever and tularemia in man. IV. The integrity of the endotoxin tolerance mechanisms during infection. J Clin Invest 1969;48:613.

REFERENCES

1. Traub R, Wisseman CL Jr. Ecological considerations in scrub typhus. I. Emerging concepts. Bull WHO 1968;39(2):209–218.

2. Traub R, Wisseman CL Jr, Ahmad N. The occurrence of scrub typhus infection in unusual habitats in West Pakistan. Trans R Soc Med Hyg 1967;61(1):23–57, 1967.

3. Traub R, Evans TM. Description of new species of Hytrichopsyllid fleas, with notes on arched pronotal combs, convergent evolution and zoogeography (Siphonaptera) Pacif. Insects 1967;9(4):603–676.

4. Traub R, Jellison WL. Evolutionary and biogeographis history and the phylogeny of vectors and reservoirs as factors in the transmission of diseases from other animals to man. In Borgdorfer W, Naacker RL, eds., Rickettsiae and Rickettsial Diseases. Proc. RML Conf. Rickettsiae and Rickettsial Diseases, Academic Press: New York, 1980, pp. 517–546.

23

INTERNATIONAL HEALTH PROGRAM 1981–1995

G. Thomas Strickland, M.D.

In 1982, I retired from the Navy to assume the Directorship of both the International Health Program (IHP) in Baltimore and the International Center for Medical Research and Training (ICMRT) (also called the PMRC) in Lahore. My career in the Navy was primarily in tropical medicine research. I trained in internal medicine at the National Naval Medical Center (NNMC) in Bethesda, and the Navy sent me to the London School of Tropical Medicine and Hygiene where I obtained an M.Sc. in clinical tropical medicine and a Ph.D. in parasitic immunology. I had extensive overseas research experiences in the Far East when I was assigned to the Naval Medical Research Unit-2 (NAMRU-2) in Taipei and during extended research ventures in Egypt. I had been director of the Navy's infectious disease research program and co-director of the Navy's infectious disease fel-

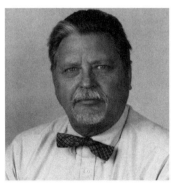

G. Thomas Strickland, M.D.

lowship and attending physician in medicine at both the NNMC and WRAMC. I was the first full-time active duty faculty member assigned to a clinical department at the Uniformed Services University of the Health Sciences (USUHS).

I had given up my laboratory at USUHS in 1981 when I edited the 6th edition of *Hunter's Tropical Medicine* and discontinued my clinical work shortly after joining the Maryland faculty in 1982. My responsibility here was to reorganize and replenish the IHP and the ICMRT at a time when both appeared to be failing. My first task would be to strengthen the ICMRT, which was hanging by a thread under the guidance of the interim director, Dr. Richard Sakai, an excellent genetic entomologist. A multitude of problems, both internal and external, had built up under the former director who left Pakistan in 1981. Relationships with the Pakistan and American authorities were at a very low point. The NIH funding had ceased, and no new sources of support were obvious. With the assistance of Dean John Dennis and Charlie Wisseman, I negotiated with USAID, both in Islamabad and in Washington, for a grant to switch the ICMRT into a facility that focused on applied research in malaria, attacking specific problems for Pakistan. At the same time, I made it known that I would pursue switching management of the ICMRT from UMAB to a nonprofit organization in Pakistan receiving scientific and technical assistance from Maryland.

This approach was initially successful, and early in 1983, the IHP was awarded a $4.3 million grant to perform community-based research in malaria. The authority of an already in place, strong local governing board was increased. The plan was to use this same group of sponsors and directors of the nongovernmental organization (NGO) who governed the ICMRT. Despite numerous difficulties, the ICMRT was able to meet some of its scientific goals. About 20 papers were published including: 1) descriptions of the malaria vectors and their bionomics in the Punjab; 2) the first documentation of chloroquine-resistant malaria in the western Indian subcontinent showing that *P. falciparum* parasites were equally resistant to amodiaquine but exquisitely sensitive to Fansidar; 3) investigations of the effects of season, weather, vector bionomics, and antimalarial drugs on malaria transmission; and 4) studies of the community epidemiology of malaria and risk factors for malaria infection and disease.

However, old prejudices, particularly with the USAID Mission in Islamabad and the Pakistan Malaria Control Program, could not be overcome, and support for the ICMRT collapsed. At that point, the goal was to keep the center open and retain as many of the well-trained Pakistani staff as possible. In July 1995, UMAB transferred the ICMRT to the Government of Pakistan, which retained about two-thirds of the staff at wages about half of that paid by the ICMRT (and less than a living wage). The facility was renamed the Pakistan Malaria Research Center (PMRC), and as far as is known, it never again performed any research. The community-based studies which had continued up until a few days before the transfer were never resumed.

Severely disappointed, I returned to Baltimore to assume my role as Director of the International Health Program on a full-time basis. I used my previous experiences and contacts to build a collaborative research program with Egyptian Universities and the Ministry of Health and NAMRU-3 in Cairo. UMAB faculty received long-term assignments to NAMRU-3 to assist their research projects. About 75 manuscripts were published by UMAB faculty working at NAMRU-3 from 1986 to 1996, including papers on schistosomiasis, amebiasis, meningitis, and abdominal tuberculosis. Dr. Peter Woodruff, the son of my professor in London and now a British psychiatrist performing research on the metabolic aspects of schizophrenia using high-resolution MRI, worked on encephalitis in Egypt and febrile illnesses in the Sudan. Emile Fox, who is currently the WHO advisor on HIV/AIDS to China, worked for four years on HIV and other infectious diseases in northeast Africa. Dr. Niel Constantine, who now directs the University Hospital's Clinical Immunology Lab, managed the NAMRU-3 Virology Division and performed extensive research on HIV, the hepatitis viruses, and other viruses. Ron Anthony, who recently retired from the School of Medicine's Pathology Department, worked on leishmaniasis in the Sudan and later went to NAMRU-2 in Indonesia where he had a three-year assignment working on malaria and HIV in Indonesia and the Philippines. Gunneal Rodier, who is currently the WHO's Director of Global Surveillance of Diseases, was assigned to NAMRU-3 for almost four years. He published about 30 papers on different aspects of HIV, hepatitis C and E, Rift valley fever, and other African infectious diseases. Jim Olson, who now is the Chief of the CDC Viral and Rickettsial Zoonoses Branch, directed the epidemiology program at NAMRU-3 for 3 years—a time when it was very productive. Another member of the IHP, Jim Murphy, also worked at NAMRU-3, although his assignment was from the University of Texas in Houston; he performed excellent work on enteric fevers and bacterial diarrheas. The Baltimore tradition at NAMRU-3 continues with Dr. Ray Arthur from the Johns Hopkins School of Hygiene & Public Health directing the Virology Division at NAMRU-3 since 1992. Dr. Arthur has collaborated extensively with the IHP and will lead the Johns Hopkins University component of an IHP-led multicenter study of hepatitis C in Egypt which started in mid-1996.

Most of my efforts in Egypt concerned collaborative research projects with different Egyptian universities and within the Egyptian Ministry of Health/USAID-sponsored Schistosomiasis Research Project. These have resulted in 35 publications on schistosomiasis, amebic liver abscess, viral hepatitis, pyrogenic meningitis, tuberculous peritonitis, and hepatic hydatid cysts. The largest part of this work was associated with an extensive countrywide random sample survey of 100,000 rural habitants for infection and morbidity due to schistosomiasis. Abdominal ultrasonography was used to screen every fifth household (25,000 subjects) for morbidity. This has been followed by assisting in WHO/Egyptian Ministry of Health/USAID-sponsored investigations of the in vitro immune responses to six candidate subunit antigens for an S. mansoni vaccine in two highly selected populations with exposures to infection. The wide use of praziquancl, a drug with excellent chemotherapeutic action with little toxicity for schistosomiasis, greatly improved this health problem in Egypt. Studies were shifted to hepatitis C (HCV) whose prevalence of infection in rural communities in the Nile delta is in the 30%–35% range. Chronic hepatitis and cirrhosis and hepatocellular carcinoma are increasing *problems* in Egypt. The IHP has been awarded a multiyear, multicenter grant to study risk factors for transmission for HCV in Egypt so that preventive procedures can be developed and applied.

Tick-transmitted bacterial infections are under study in Maryland. UMAB has a grant to study the outcomes of antibiotic therapy of Lyme disease. This grant supports the Lyme disease registry at the State Health Department. The data set of over

1,600 Lyme disease cases is the most complete available and provides opportunities for descriptive papers of Lyme disease, for risk factor assessment, and for investigating outcomes of antibiotic therapy. In addition, my group has investigated and reported outbreaks of Lyme disease in a summer camp on the Eastern Shore and the first cases of human monocytic ehrlichiosis in Maryland. Future directions of research will evaluate the effects of global toxins on endemic infectious diseases.

PERTINENT REFERENCES BY FACULTY MEMBERS

Abdel-Wahab MF, Esmat G, Farrag A, El-Boraey YA, Strickland GT. Grading of hepatic schistosomiasis by the use of ultrasonography. Am J Trop Med Hyg 1992;46:403–408.

Abdel-Wahab MF, Esmat G, Farrag A, El-Boraey YA, Strickland GT. Ultrasonographic prediction of esophageal varices in schistosomiasis mansoni. Am J Gastroenterol 1993;88:560–563.

Abdel-Wahab MF, Esmat G, Milad M, Abdel-Razek S, Strickland GT. Characteristic sonographic pattern of schistosomal hepatic filbrosis. Am J Trop Med Hyg 1989;40:72–76.

Abdel-Wahab MF, Esmat G, Narooz SI, Yosery A, Struewing JP, Strickland GT. Sonographic studies of school children in a village endemic for *S. mansoni*. Trans R Soc Trop Med Hyg 1990;84:69–73.

Abdel-Wahab MF, Esmat G, Ramzy I, Fouad R, Abdel-Rahman M, Yosery A, Strickland GT. Schistosoma haematobium infection in Egyptian school children: Demonstration of both hepatic and urinary tract morbidity by ultrasonography. Trans R Soc Trop Med Hyg 1992; 86:406–409.

Abdel-Wahab MF, Ramzy I, Esmat G, El Kafass H, Strickland GT. Ultrasound for detecting *Schistosoma haematobium* urinary tract complications: comparison with radiographic procedures. J Urol 1992; 48:346–350.

Abdel-Wahab MF, Strickland GT. Abdominal ultrasonography for assessing morbidity from schistosomiasis: 2. Hospital studies. Trans R Soc Trop Med Hyg 1993;87:135–137.

Abdel-Wahab MF, Yosery A, Narooz S, Esmat G, El Hak S, Nasif S, Strickland GT. Is *S. mansoni* replacing *S. haematobium* in the Fayoum? Am J Trop Med Hyg 1993;49:697–700.

Abdel-Wahab MF, Zakaria S, Kamel M, Abdel-Khaliq MK, Mabrouk MA, Esmat G, Thomas DL, Strickland GT. High seroprevalence of hepatitis C infection among risk groups in Egypt. Am J Trop Med Hyg 1994;51:563–567.

Ahmed L, El Rooby A, Zakaria S, Strickland GT. Ultrasonography in the diagnosis and management of 52 patients with amebic liver abscess in Cairo. Rev Infect Dis 1990;12:330–337.

Ahmed L, Zadaria S, El Rooby A, Strickland GT. Ultrasonographic resolution time for amebic liver abscess. Am J Top Med Hyg 1989;41:406–410.

Bassily S, Strickland GT, Abdel-Wahab MF, Esmat GE, Narooz S, El Masry NA, Cosntantine NT, Struewing JP. Efficacy of hepatitis B vaccination in primary school children from a village endemic for *S. mansoni*. J Infect Dis 1992;166:265–268.

Browning MD, Narooz SI, Strickland GT, El-Masry NA, Abdel-Wahab MF. Clinical characteristics and response to therapy in Egyptian children infected with schistosoma haematobium. J Infect Dis 1984; 149:998–1004.

Coyle BS, Strickland GT, Liang YY, McCarter R, Israel E. The public health impact of Lyme disease in Maryland. J Infect Dis 1996; 173:1260–1262.

Fox E, Khaliq AA, Sarwar M, Strickland GT. Chloroquine resistant Plasmodium falciparum: Now in Pakistani Punjab. Lancet 1985;1: 1432–1435.

Fox E, Strickland GT, Sarwar M, Shamim M, Zafa-Latif A, Khaliq AA. Reliable assessment of malaria prevalence through village clinics. Trans R Soc Trop Med Hyg 1987;81:115–117.

Fox E, Strickland GT. La recherche medical Luxembourgeoise: Use alternative de cooperation avec les pays en development? Le Corps Med 1986;27:957–960.

Fox E, Strickland GT. The interrelationship of Plasmodium falciparum and Plasmodium vivax in the Punjab. Trans R Soc Trop Med Hyg 1989;83:471–473.

Ghabrah TM, Strickland GT, Tsarev S, Yarbough P, Farci P, Engle R, Emerson S, Purcell R. Acute viral hepatitis in Saudia Arabia: Seroepidemiologic analysis, risk factors, clinical manifestations and evidence for a sixth hepatitis agent. Clin Infect Dis 1995; 21:621–627.

Ghaffar YA, Fattah SA, Kamel M, Badr R, Mahomed FF, Strickland GT. The impact of endemic schistosomiasis on acute viral hepatitis. Am J Trop Med Hyg 1991;45:743–750.

Ghaffar YA, Kamel M, El-Sobky M, Bahnasy R, Strickland GT. Response to hepatitis B vaccine in infants born to mothers with schistosomiasis. Lancet 1989;2:272.

Hadi H, Fox E, Strickland GT, Pervez M, Chowdhry MA. Endemic malaria in Punjabi children: a diagnostic challenge. Pak J Med Res 1985;24:63–68.

Hammad TA, Abdel-Wahab MF, DeClaris N, El-Sahly A, El-Kady N, Strickland GT. Comparative evaluation of the use of artificial neural networks for modeling the epidemiology of schistosomiasis mansoni. Trans R Soc Trop Med Hyg 1996;90:372–376.

Kandil MR, Farraq A-K F, El-Rehawy MS, Tarkhan MA, Rashwan NM, Zarzour AH, Khalil M, Strickland GT. Pyrogenic meningitis in Assiut, Egypt. Infect Dis Clin Pract 1992;2:202–211.

Khaliq AA, Fox E, Sarwar M, Strickland GT. Amodiaquine fails to cure chloroquine resistant Plasmodium falciparum in the Punjab. Trans R Soc Trop Med Hyg 1987;81:157–159.

Khaliq AA, Fox E, Strickland GT, Zafar-Latif A, Chowdhry MA. Malaria in a rural Punjabi community: High infection rates with low prevalence of disease. Pak J Med Res 1985;24:69–74.

Khaliq AA, Sarwar M, Fox E, Strickland GT. Chloroquine resistant Plasmodium falciparum in the Punjab. Pak J Med Res 1985;24: 89–93.

Madwar MA, El Tahawy M, Strickland GT. The relationship between uncomplicated schistosomiasis and hepatitis B infection. Trans R Soc Trop Med Hyg 1989;83:233–236.

Madwar MA, Hassan MH, Strickland GT. Circulating antigens for assessing cure in schistosomiasis mansoni. Trans R Soc Trop Med Hyg 1988;82:881–884.

Madwar MA, Strickland GT, El-Ridi AM, Aboul-Magd LA, Mourad AA, Hassan MM. Circulating antigens in diagnosis and assessment of cure in Bilharziasis. Afro-Arab Liver J 1988;1:69–76.

Medhat A, Abdel-Aty MA, Nafeh M, Hamman H, Abdel-Samia A, Strickland GT. Foci of *Schistosoma mansoni* in Assuit Province in Middle Egypt. Trans R Soc Trop Med Hyg 1993;87:404–405.

Nafeh MA, Medhat A, Abdul-Hameed A-G, Ahmad YA, Rashwan NM, Strickland GT. Tuberculous peritonitis in Egypt: the value of laparoscopy in diagnosis. Am J Trop Med Hyg 1992;47:470–477.

Nafeh MA, Medhat A, Swifae Y, Moftah FM, Mohamed A, Soliman A-G A, Strickland GT. Ultrasonographic changes of the liver in schistosoma haematobium infection. Am J Trop Med Hyg 1992;46: 225–230.

Peña C, Woubeshett M, Grigor JK, Stickland GT. Lyme disease surveillance in Maryland: Sources and outcomes of suspected cases. J Spirochetal Tickborne Dis 1996;3:159–164.

Prevez M, Macdonald M, Fox E, Strickland GT, Hassan H, Chowdhry MA. Malaria transmission assessed by infant smear surveys compared to entomological techniques. Pak J Med Res 1985;24:81–84.

Salama H, Abdel-Wahab MF, Strickland GT. Diagnosis and treatment of hepatic hydatid cyst with aid of echo-guided percutaneous cyst puncture. Clin Infect Dis 1995;21:1372–1376.

Shamin, M., Strickland GT, Fox E, Chowdhry MA. Clinic malaria smear surveys as a determinant of malaria prevalence. Pak J Med Res 1985;24:75–78.

Steinberg SH, Strickland GT, Pena C, Israel E. Lyme disease surveillance in Maryland, 1992. Ann Epidemiol 1996;6:24-29.

Strickland GT, Mohydin MAZ. Malaria in the Punjab. Pak J Med Res 1985;24:49–52.

Strickland GT, Abdel-Wahab MF. Abdominal ultrasonography for assessing morbidity from schistosomiasis: 1. Community studies. Trans R Soc Trop Med Hyg 1993;87:132–134.

Strickland GT, Abdel-Wahab MF. Schistosomiasis on the Aswan High Dam Lake. Egypt J Bilharz 1990;12:197–205.

Strickland GT, Caisley I, Woubeshet M, Israel E. Antibiotic therapy for Lyme disease in Maryland. Public Health Rep 1994;109: 745–749.

Strickland GT, Fox E, Hadi H. Malaria and splenomegaly in the Punjab. Trans R Soc Trop Med Hyg 1988;82:667–670.

Strickland GT, Fox E, Sarwar M, Khaliq AA, and Macdonald M. Effects of chloroquine, amodiaquine and pyrimethamine-sulfadoxine on Plasmodium falciparum gametocytes. Am J Trop Med Hyg 1986;35: 259–262.

Strickland GT, Hoffman SL. Strategies for control for malaria. Sci Am:Sci Med 1994;1:24–33, 1994.

Strickland GT, Khaliq AA, Sarwar M, Hadi H, Pervez M, Fox E. Effects of FANSIDAR on chloroquine resistant Plasmodium falciparum in Pakistan. Am J Trop Med Hyg 1986;35:61–65.

Strickland GT, Trivedi L, Watkins S, et al: Cluster of Lyme disease cases at a summer camp in Kent County, Maryland. Emerg Infect Dis 1996;2:44–46.

Strickland GT, Zarar-Latif A, Fox E, Khaliq AA, Chowdhry MA. Endemic malaria in four villages of the Pakistani province of Punjab. Trans R Soc Trop Med Hyg 1987;81:36–41.

Strickland GT. Fever in the returned traveler. Med Clin North Am 1992;76:1375–1392.

Strickland GT. Malaria: Old knowledge and new developments. Ann Saudi Med 1987;7:3–11.

Strickland GT. Tropical infection of the gastrointestinal tract and liver series. Gastrointestinal manifestations of schistosomiasis. Gut 1994;35:1334–1337.

Jung PI, Nahas JN, Strickland GT, McCarter R, Israel I. Maryland physician's survey on Lyme disease. Md Med J 1994;43:447–450.

Strickland GT. Prevalence of hepatitis B surface antigenemia among patients with *Schistosoma mansoni*. Ann Saudi Med 1994;14:263.

Waked IA, Saleh SM, Moustafa MS, Raouf AA, Thomas DL, Strickland GT. High prevalence of hepatitis C in Egyptian patients with chronic liver disease. Gut 1995;36:111–113.

Zafar-Latif A, Strickland GT, Fox E, Khaliq AA, Chowdhry MA. Seasonal fluctuation of malaria in four selected villages of the Punjab. Pak J Med Res 1985;24:53–61.

24

PRODUCTIVE COLLABORATION BETWEEN THE SCHOOL OF MEDICINE AND THE MILITARY SERVICES

Theodore E. Woodward, M.D.

At mid-20th century, after World War II, various medical schools found it expedient to reshape their educational and research programs in order to keep abreast of numerous medical advances. Many medical professionals had gained new experiences and capabilities in preventive medicine (epidemiology) and in diseases of global and tropical significance which were, or could be, threats to the United States. Dr. H.C. Byrd was President of the University of Maryland, and served under an active Board of Regents. An early charge from College Park was a directive that clinical departments of the medical school be headed by full-time professors. This led to the system of geographical full-time faculty members, which meant that they were to receive a base salary and be allowed an overpractice income derived from private patients examined in the hospital proper. Salaries were determined by the medical dean and administrative authorities. These new guidelines led to extensive changes in medical school and hospital activities, some of which are described in the preceding chapters.

MARYLAND'S MILITARY
CONNECTION: A JOINT RELATIONSHIP

Traditionally, the medical school has been associated intimately with the United States Military Services. These associations will be briefly described. Dr. William A. Hammond, Professor of Anatomy and Physiology at the medical school from 1859 to 1861, was appointed Surgeon General of the United States Army in 1862 during the Civil War, at age 34. By special order, he helped create the Army Medical Museum in 1862 which became the Armed Forces Institute of Pathology (AFIP), a leading pathologic center in the world. Also, he helped organize a rapid system for removing wounded from the battlefield and ultimate hospitalization. Perhaps this could be considered as

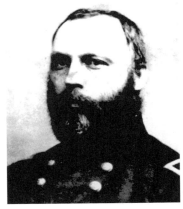

William A. Hammond, M.D., Professor, Anatomy and Physiology, 1859–1861; Surgeon General U.S. Army, 1862–1864

a suggested forerunner of the Shock Trauma Unit, initiated at Maryland by Dr. R Adams Cowley, a century later.

In the early 20th century, Dr. Arthur M. Shipley (a 1902 graduate) had a distinguished WW I record as Chief Surgeon of the 8th Evacuation Hospital in France. With his unit was Dr. W. Houston Toulson, a graduate in 1912, who later became Head of Urology at Maryland, and a leading Baltimore urologist. Dr. Shipley was Chief of Surgery at the University of Maryland hospital from 1920 to 1948, and established an outstanding training and practice program.

Dr. Norman T. Kirk, a 1910 graduate of the medical school, was a noted surgeon appointed Surgeon General of the United States Army in 1943 during WW II. He became a proponent for guillotine amputation for battlefield in-

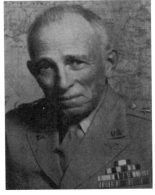

Norman T. Kirk, M.D., Surgeon General U.S. Army, 1943–1947

juries and devised the operation currently known as Kirk's amputation below the knee.

Two deans of the medical school who came to Maryland in this high position after their military retirements were Dr. Robert U. Patterson, Dean from 1943 to 1946, and Dr. William S. Stone, Dean from 1955 to 1969. They were Surgeon General, U.S. Army, and Commandant, Walter Reed Army Medical Center, respectively. Their capabilities as educators and administrators greatly enhanced the efficiency of many new academic programs. They established firm and productive relationships with University authorities at College Park, where final administrative decisions were made with approval of the Board of Regents. Dr. Stone's vision and capabilities regarding battlefield injuries obtained during the Korean War helped place the University in an enviable position. This ultimately led to development of the Shock Trauma Unit under Dr. Cowley's direction. The original funds were obtained from the Department of Defense. Major assistance during the early stages of this unique unit was provided by Dr. George Yeager and Dr. Arlie Mansberger, each of whom had gained valuable military experiences involving battlefield trauma during WW II.

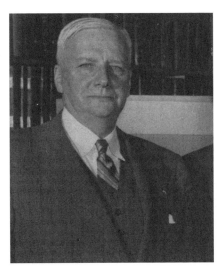

Robert V. Patterson, M.D., Surgeon General U.S. Army; Dean, 1943–1946

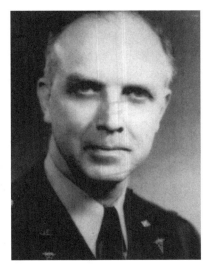

William S. Stone, M.D., Commandant WRAIR; Dean, 1955–1969

The WW II years provided opportunities for civilian physicians to broaden their capability of clinical surgery and medicine through exposure of the American soldier to traumatic wounds, pestilential, and emotional hazards—all thoroughly foreign to them under ordinary circumstances. Drs. Maurice C. Pincoffs, Louis Krause, George H. Yeager, Monte Edwards, Frank Geraghty, Lewis Gundry, Harry Hull, Vernon Langluttig, and William S. Love were senior faculty members whose leadership roles merit special recognition. The University of Maryland Hospital physicians formed the 42nd General Hospital which rendered exemplary service in the Southwest Pacific area, India, and the Philippine Islands.

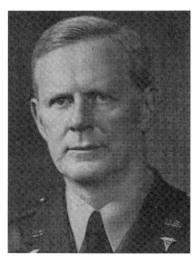

Maurice C. Pincoffs, M.D., Chairman, Department of Medicine, 1922–1954

Initially organized as one hospital unit, it split into two separate general hospitals with smaller advanced surgical groups for work in combat areas. Drs. Pincoffs, Yeager, and Edwards commanded these units. Later Dr. Pincoffs (Col.) was appointed Chief Preventive Medicine Officer under General Douglas A. MacArthur. Col. Pincoffs planned and personally participated in the initial field study which demonstrated conclusively that atabrine was a most effective antimalarial agent when taken daily.

Among the large cadre of younger Baltimore physicians assigned to the 42nd General Hospital, or to other overseas branches of the military medical services were Drs. William Helfrich, Kennedy Waller, Edward F. Cotter, Ernest I. Cornbrooks, Harry Bowie, Everett Diggs, Ephraim T. Lisansky, Carl Bailey, Irving Freeman, Harry M. Robinson, Jr., James R. Karns, Edward Muller, Samuel T. R. Revell, Jr., Timothy Callahan, John Z. Bowers, Theodore E. Woodward, and others.

Drs. Ernest I. Cornbrooks, Jr. and John Albrittain, each graduates of the class of 1935, had distinguished careers in the United States Navy during World War II. After their Chief Residencies at the University Hospital in Gynecology and Obstetrics,

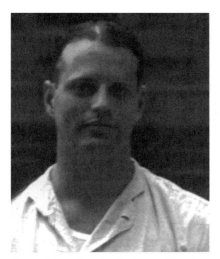
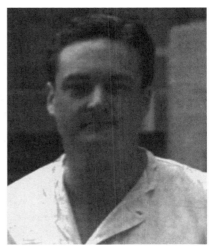

Ernest I. Cornbrooks, Jr., Class of 1935,
Cmdr. U.S. Navy

John Albrittain, M.D., Class of 1935,
Deputy Surgeon General U.S. Navy

respectively, they entered the military service during the war. Dr. Cornbrooks served in the U.S. Navy and Marines in the European and Pacific theatres and achieved the rank of Commander. Throughout this service, three combat ships on which he served were sunk by enemy action. After the war he became one of Baltimore's leading gynecologists and taught for a number of years at the medical school and hospital. Dr. John Albrittain's service during WW II was equally impressive. He remained in the Naval Service as a Line Officer and became Deputy Surgeon General.

After the war, a close relationship continued with the viral and rickettsial diseases unit at the Walter Reed Medical Research Center. Dr. Woodward spent every Thursday afternoon there working with Dr. Joseph E. Smadel and others while establishing a private medical practice in Baltimore. Research work on the rickettsial diseases, tularemia, brucellosis, and meningitis continued. During this period in 1948, successful antibiotic trials with chloramphenicol for scrub typhus and typhoid fever were performed in Malaya under a Department of Defense contract. This was the *first* off-campus contract grant to the University of Maryland and to the Department of Medicine for a total amount of $50,000. Biologic warfare defense research activities developed a little later with basic work performed at WRAIR, USAMRIID (Fort Detrick), and in Baltimore. Annual research grants and long-term general contracts followed for support of the laboratory work and the vaccine volunteer trials at the Jessup Maryland House of Correction and a special ward at the University Hospital. These were large grant funds needed to support all activities such as salaries of investigators, fellows, technicians, secretaries, travel, and overhead expenses. Beginning in 1950, millions of dollars were provided for research which extended over three decades. Other fund sources included grants-in-aid by pharmaceutical firms for special antimicrobial studies. Hence, the medical school and hospital were very actively involved in helping develop new knowledge of serious infectious diseases, including plague, all rickettsioses, as well as important new data regarding pathogenesis and defense measures for biologic warfare agents. That threat was a definite reality.

Dr. Woodward contributed to the Armed Forces Epidemiological Board's (AFEB) programs first as a member of the Commission on Epidemiological Survey from 1952 to 1973, and as its Director from 1959 to 1973. He was a member of the Commission on Rickettsial Diseases from 1955 to 1973, and an associate member of the Commission on Immunization from 1950 to 1973. He served a long tenure as president of the AFEB from 1976 to 1978 and 1980 to 1990, when many important collaborative problems on infectious diseases were under study at Maryland on pathogenesis and vaccine protection.

James (Jim) Nuttall, class of 1939, took a two-year rotating internship at the University Hospital followed by a year in Preventive Medicine at Johns Hopkins School of Hygiene and Public Health. He joined the Air Force as a flight surgeon over Germany and Southern Europe (Balkans). After the war, Dr. Nuttall progressed through the ranks to Brigadier General and directed the important aerospace program in San Antonio. He retired to his home in Plaza Del Ray, California.

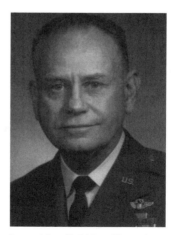

James Nuttall, M.D., Class of 1939, Brig. Gen. USAF; Director Aerospace Program

Col. John Rizzolo, class of 1938, contributed importantly to the United States Air Force (USAF) as Head of

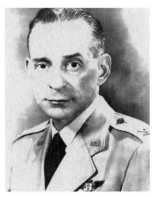

John Rizzolo, M.D., Class of 1938; Head Preventive Medicine USAF, 1959; Deputy Director AFEB, 1959–1961

Preventive Medicine (1959), and later as Executive Secretary of the Armed Forces Epidemiological Board (1959–1961). After his retirement, he was Research Administrator of the American Cancer Society.

Richard Worthington, M.D., class of 1938, chose the U.S. Navy for his career after service during the war. He was appointed to the rank of Rear Admiral.

Frederick W. Plugge IV, M.D., a 1957 graduate, served his internship at the Royal Victoria Hospital, Montreal, and residency in surgery at the University of Maryland, 1958–1962. As a Reserve Officer in the United States Air Force, he gained further surgical experience in England, Germany, California, and other Air Force centers. From 1968 to 1978, he was Chief of General

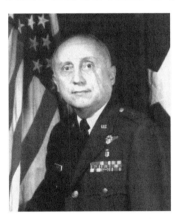

Brig. Gen. Frederick W. Plugge IV, M.D., Class of 1957

Surgery, and later, Chairman of the Department of Surgery at the Andrews Air Force Base. He commanded Air Force hospitals in Weisbaden (1978–1981) and the Travers Air Force Base (1981–1988).

While he was Director of Medical Inspection at the USAF Inspection and Safety Center (1985–1988), his contributions greatly improved medical, dental, and surgical procedure practices, improved management accountability, war time medical preparedness, and peace time medical performance. Dr. Plugge, during his distinguished military career, received numerous citations and awards. In July 1987, he was promoted to Brigadier General USAF. He retired in 1991 and settled in Chevy Chase, Maryland.

Dr. William D. Tigertt (Brigadier General, USA), former Commandant of WRAIR and USAMRIID (Fort Detrick) came to Maryland in 1972 as Professor of Medicine and Pathology to di-

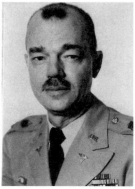

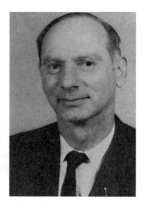

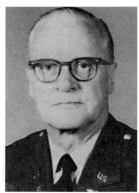

William T. Tigertt, M.D.   *Abram S. Benenson, M.D.*   *Dan Crozier, M.D.*

rect the hospital's clinical laboratories. He served most effectively. His colleagues Col. Abram Benenson and Col. Dan Crozier joined as adjunct faculty members. Their broad knowledge of potential biologic offensive agents and epidemiology greatly enhanced the overall program in infectious diseases.

James J. Cerda, M.D., graduated from the medical school in 1961, and from 1962 to 1964, he was a medical resident at the University Hospital. Previously, from 1951 to 1954, he served in the U.S. Navy, and contributed actively to the U.S. Naval Reserve, 1958–1990. He became a Rear Admiral, M.C., of the U.S. Naval Reserve, now retired. Dr. Cerda settled at the University of Florida, Gainesville, where he is Professor of Medicine and Gastroenterology. He is an authority on the nutritional aspects of gastrointestinal disorders.

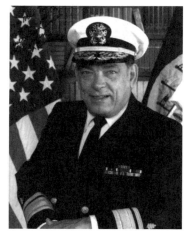

With this collaborative military-civilian program, the Department of Medicine grew and flourished. With it, the University profited through the enrichment, enthusiasm, and help of new and vigorous personnel. All of this enabled Maryland to achieve and en-

James J. Cerda, M.D., Class of 1961, Rear Admiral USNR (Ret.); Professor of Medicine, University of Florida

hance its stature. Drs. Merrill J. Snyder, Richard B. Hornick, Frank M. Calia, Morton I. Rapoport, Leonard Morse, Sheldon E. Greisman, Charles L. Wisseman, Jr., George Entwisle, William S. Spicer, Robert Traub, Herbert Barnett, and Ted Alevizatos are former faculty members who came to Maryland with a military connection. Even the cholera and enteric diseases vaccine program including *E. coli* and *Shigella* studies were government oriented by way of the Department of Defense and the National Institutes of Health. Dr. Myron Levine and his remarkable group represent fulfillment of the earlier collaboration attributed to a Walter Reed, Fort Detrick, NIH, and the Maryland team program. The medical school, the military, and the public profited equally. We can be very proud of these intermarriages which did not provoke any genetic abnormalities. All participants became leaders in their respective fields.

Perhaps it is appropriate to close by commenting that over the last two centuries, society has witnessed remarkable advances in the field of infectious diseases that have improved life expectancy from about age 40 in the early 1800s to age 78 at the end of the 20th century. During those years, epidemic scourges such as yellow fever, typhus, typhoid fever, smallpox, cholera, malaria, and tuberculosis literally wiped out populations and caused panic in those who survived. Infectious diseases have not been eradicated, nor is that ever likely to happen.

Advances in medical practice, education, and research have played significant roles in elevating standards in Baltimore, Maryland, the United States, and abroad. Baltimore has enjoyed and contributed to this rich heritage of progress, which has continued from its earliest beginnings in colonial America and sustained itself to 2000. Faculty members of the University of Maryland School of Medicine and Hospital can be proud. These achievements coupled with those of its illustrious sister institution, the Johns Hopkins University School of Medicine and Hospital, have benefited the citizens of the city and state and helped maintain Baltimore's posture as a leading American medical center.

Those first and significant contributions to the detection, prevention, and cure of important infectious diseases by health professionals made at the medical school and hospital at Lombard and Greene Streets during the past two centuries are proudly given their due recognition (see the following Infectious Diseases Time Line).

INFECTIOUS DISEASES TIME LINE
(Bold indicates activity occurring outside of the University of Maryland.)

1796	**Edward Jenner introduced vaccination for smallpox**
1800	**First introduction (with Waterhouse) of smallpox vaccination in America**
1811	Early prediction of the relationship between insects and diseases
1833	First medical school course on preventive medicine in America
1842	First systematic monograph on febrile illness in America
1878	Original treatise on leprosy in Baltimore
1879	First description of erysipelatous pneumonia
1882	**Koch identified specific agent, mycobacterium tuberculosis**
1883	Confirmation that gonorrhea is a bacterial disease
1894	First description of blastomycosis
1906	First description of a new disease, histoplasmosis
1909	First treatise on rabies in Maryland
1938	Initial detection and clinical report of disseminated histoplasmosis (Darling's disease) in Maryland
1947	Development of new simplified technique for cultivation of tubercle bacilli

ENTERIC DISEASES

Typhoid Fever

1800	**Eberth described typhoid bacillus**
1896	**Widal test for sero diagnoses of typhoid reported**
1948	Reported first known specific cure of typhoid fever
1950, 1983	First effective use of glucocorticoids which greatly reduced mortality in critically ill typhoid patients
1961, 1969, 1970	Established the human infectious dose of *Salmonella typhosa*-based IB classic studies in volunteers. this basic information set the stage for evaluation of vaccine efficacy
1975–1977, 1992	Long-term studies in volunteers clarified the limited efficacy of conventional typhoid vaccines (phenol and acetone inactivated). First use and report of

markedly improved protection with genetically manipulated vaccines given orally

Asiatic Cholera

1884   **Robert Koch identified *V. cholerae***
1960   Original demonstration that the intestinal mucosa is histologically intact in cholera patients. This observation refuted the long-held views of Virchow (1879) and Koch (1884) that the intestinal epithelium was desquamated. This important finding suggested that the pathologic lesion was biochemical and that a toxin was responsible for the physiologic abnormalities and diarrhea which characterize cholera. Contribution, with others, that oral rehydration of cholera patiients which greatly simplified treatment of this epidemic disorder and established the oral infectious human dose of *Vibrio cholerae* which was essential for the planning, better understanding, and interpretation of vaccine field trials
1975, 1988 Developed and tested the first effective genetically manipulated viable vaccines useful for prevention of cholera

Bacillary Dysentery

1971   First human testing of viable hybrid vaccines given orally which showed marked protection against bacillary dysentery

Protective Effect of Gastric Acid

1971   First convincing demonstration that gastric acid influences pathogenesis and is an effective barrier to infection caused by *Vibro cholerae* and *Salmonella typhosa*

Rickettsial Diseases

1906   **Ricketts incriminated ticks and transmitted Rocky Mountain spotted fever to animals**
1930   Report of index case of murine typhus fever which led to rickettsial isolation from rats and fleas

1941	Initial reported case of murine typhus fever in Jamaica, B.W.I.
1944	First report of studies in volunteers in an endemic area of epidemic typhus that one large dose of vaccine protects against active infection
1948, 1950	First known specific therapeutic cures: scrub typhus fever, Rocky Mountain spotted fever, murine typhus fever
1949, 1952	First use of antibiotics for chemoprophylaxis of scrub typhus based on classic field studies in volunteers
1952, 1954	First isolation of viable rickettsia from patients convalescent from scrub typhys and Rocky Mountain spotted fever. These findings confirmed concepts of long-term microbial persistence
1952	First to determine the human infectious dose of *Coxiella burnetii* (Q fever) in volunteers and showed that vaccines protect against illness after aerosol exposure with pathogenic viable Q fever Rickettsia
1968	Development of zoogeographic phylogenetic, evolutionary, and geologic factors and a hypothesis of "ecological islands" and "oases of infection" to account for and correctly predict the distribution of some ecto parasite-borne infections in various parts of the world, including habitats of South Asia and Africa (chigger-borne rickettsioses, plaque, tularemia, etc.)
1972	It was shown in volunteers that conventional vaccines for Rocky Mountain spotted fever did not protect against infection
1976	First immediate demonstration of *R. rickettsiae* in skin tissues of patients with Rocky Mountain spotted fever by immune fluorescence technique
1977	First report that the agent of Rocky Mountain spotted fever can be transmitted to humans by blood transfusion

Malaria

1973, 1975	Early studies of induced malaria in humans and first demonstration in volunteers that an attenuated

sporozoite vaccine is protective for *P. falciparum* infection

Measles

1961   First confirmation that an attenuated live measles vaccine protects children against active infection and induces immunity

1964   Development of a simple, easily reproducible, inexpensive method for the serologic identification of measles infection and an immune response to measles vaccine

Pyrogenic Meningitis

1951, 1953   With the advent of chloramphenicol and Aureomycin, the first two broad-spectrum antibiotics, it was initially shown that either were very effective when given solely for treatment of patients with meningitis caused by hemophilus influenzae and in those caused by meningococci (chloramphenicol) and pneumococci (chloramphenicol). When given by the oral route, their use greatly simplified treatment in remote areas, i.e., one drug given orally.

Plague

1665   **Plague of London**
1894   **Plague bacillus identified, Yersin, Kitasato**
1952, 1953   First demonstration that the broad-spectrum antibiotics, chloramphenicol and tetramycin, given orally rapidly cure the septicemic and pneumonic types of human plague. This greatly simplified treatment in remote endemic areas.

Tularemia

1949, 1950   Report of first specific cures of experimentally induced tularemia in animals with Aureomycin and chloramphenicol. First report of human therapeutic cures with these antibiotics given orally. First demonstration in humans that immunization against tularemia can be accomplished safely using an aerosolized living attenuated vaccine. Vaccination by this route is accompanied only by a mild self-limiting infection and induces immunity equal to or better than the standard acupunture method.

Nosocomial Infections

1978   Pioneering study and report of the importance of hospital-acquired infections and recommendations for an organized data reporting system

Yellow Fever

1793   First rebuttal to the concept that yellow fever is contagious

1797   First published statement by a physician that yellow fever is not contagious

1800   Napoleon sells Louisiana to Jefferson because of yellow fever epidemic

1900   Reed Commission: mosquito transmission of yellow fever, viral etiology

1900   First experimentally induced case of yellow fever (with Reed Commission)

Fever

1991   First comprehensive monograph on fever since Wunderlich, in 1868, describing its significance, characterization, mediators, pathogenesis, methods of detection, and management. In a later carefully controlled and balanced study, it was shown that the body temperature of healthy adults is 95.0°–99.9° and not 98.6°.

ADDITIONAL HISTORIC LANDMARKS

1876   **Anthrax bacillus discovered by Pasteur and Koch**
1883   **Phagocytosis described by Metchnikoff**
1890   **Kitasato and Yersin describe antitoxin**
1910   **Ehrlich discovers salvarsan; describes antibodies**
1929   **Fleming discovers penicillin; Florey-chain further developed, demonstrated specific action**

| 1944 | Avery, MacLeod, and McCarthy report the biologic activity of DNA |
| 1948 | Introduction of broad-spectrum antibiotics |

Conquest of Infectious Diseases

First Contributions of New Medical Knowledge by University of Maryland Faculty Members

ENTERIC DISEASES

TYPHOID FEVER

Reported First known specific cure of Typhoid Fever in 1948

First effective use of glucocorticoids which greatly reduced mortality in critically ill typhoid patients

Developed a model volunteer studies program

Established the human infectious dose of salmonella typhosa based on classic studies in volunteers; this basic information set the stage for evaluation of vaccine efficacy.

First demonstration in volunteers that the toxic clinical manifestations of typhoid fever are not caused by circulating endotoxin. This provided better clarification of pathogenesis and management, 1961.

Long term studies in volunteers proved the limited efficacy of conventional typhoid vaccines (phenol and acetone inactivated).

Several years later new laboratory investigation and extended volunteer studies showed markedly improved protection with genetically manipulated vaccines given orally 1975, 1976, 1977.

First convincing demonstration that gastric acid influences pathogenesis and is an effective barrier to infection caused by vibrio cholerae and salmonella typhosa

ASIATIC CHOLERA

Original demonstration that the intestinal mucosa is histologically intact in cholera patients. This observation refuted the long-held views of Virchow (1879) and Koch (1884) that the intestinal epithelium was desquamated or flayed.

This important finding suggested that the pathologic lesion was biochemical and that a toxin was responsible for the physiologic abnormalities and diarrhea which characterize cholera.

Contribution, with others, to oral rehydration of cholera patients which greatly simplified treatment of this epidemic disorder

Established the oral infectious human dose of vibrio cholerae which was essential for planning, better understanding, and interpretations of vaccine field trials

Developed and tested the first effective genetically manipulated viable vaccines useful for prevention of cholera

BACILLARY DYSENTERY

First human testing of viable hybrid vaccines given orally which showed marked protection against bacillary dysentery.